# A Colour Atlas of
# NURSING PROCEDURES
## in Accidents & Emergencies

**John B. Bache,** FRCS(Ed)
Consultant in Accident & Emergency Department
Leighton Hospital, Crewe, England

**Carolyn R. Armitt,** SRN
Sister in Accident & Emergency Department
Leighton Hospital, Crewe, England

**J. Ruth Tobiss,** SRN
Sister in Accident & Emergency Department
Leighton Hospital, Crewe, England

**Wolfe Medical Publications Ltd**

# Contents

| *Procedure* | *Page* |
|---|---|

# Introduction

Each procedure described in this Atlas is complete in itself. Certain cross-references are inevitable but, in order to avoid the necessity of turning the pages backwards and forwards repeatedly, we have allowed ourselves a fair degree of repetition.

In common with many hospitals, the Central Sterile Supply Department of Leighton Hospital produces pre-packed sets – for dressings, suturings or knee aspirations, for instance – the full contents of which are listed whenever used. They may include certain items which are not always required but which could be needed during the course of the procedure and, therefore, should be readily available. For various reasons, it is not always possible for procedures to be absolutely sterile when performed in the Accident and Emergency Department but it is essential that they should be as aseptic as possible.

A major problem was to decide which procedures to include and which to omit. We have limited ourselves to those which are commonly undertaken by nursing staff in a typical Accident and Emergency Department and those which, although performed by medical staff, also involve nurses. Clearly a number of procedures described are performed throughout a hospital.

There are obviously many variations for almost all of the procedures included in this Atlas. The methods described are those used routinely in this hospital and we believe them to be universally acceptable, although alternatives are available and commonly used elsewhere. In general, the sizes referred to in the text are suitable for an average-sized adult man.

Any treatment must be preceded by an explanation to the patient in order to reassure him. It is also important that the appropriate observations (such as temperature, pulse and blood pressure) are recorded before, during or after many of the procedures.

At the conclusion of every treatment, if the patient is being discharged from hospital, the nurse should ensure that analgesia and/or antibiotics are available if required. Similarly, she should check that the patient is given clear instructions concerning exercises, when treatment is to be discontinued and whether he is to return to hospital.

# 1 Cervical collar

## Uses
1 Injuries of the cervical spine, including whiplash injuries.
2 Torticollis.
3 Cervical spondylosis.

## Equipment
a) Foam rubber cervical collar of suitable size, covered with cotton tubular bandage.
b) Scissors.

## Procedure
1 Expose the neck and remove jewellery.
2 With the patient looking straight ahead, position the collar under the chin.
3 Cut a 1cm hole in one of the collar ties, just to one side of the foam rubber.
4 Thread the other tie through the hole (Figure 1) and fasten under the chin.
5 Ensure that the collar fits snugly under the chin.
6 The collar ties may require to be trimmed with scissors. (Figure 2)

## Advice to patients
The collar may be removed for washing.
Follow the doctor's instructions regarding how long the collar should be worn, and whether or not it should be worn at night.

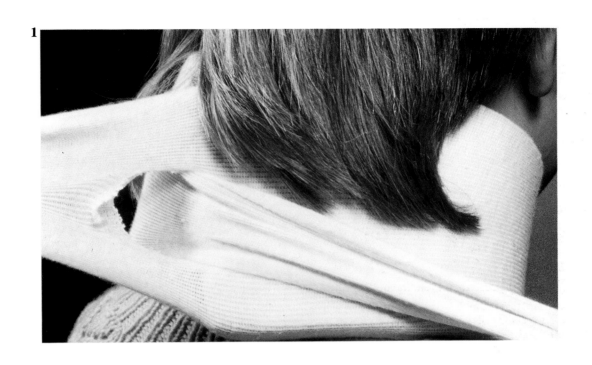

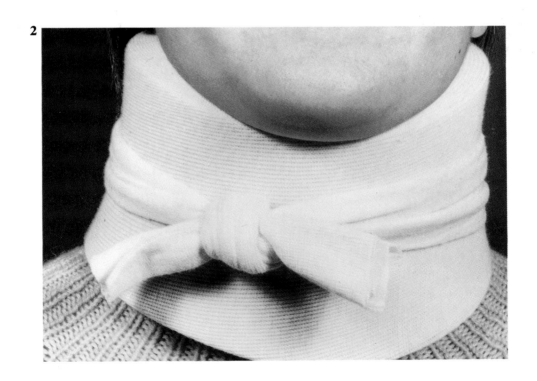

## 2 Elasticated tubular support: (A) to the elbow

### Uses
1 Joint effusions and sprains.
2 Soft tissue injuries.
3 Following aspiration of the joint or a bursa.
4 Following removal of Plaster of Paris.

### Equipment
*a)* Elasticated tubular support, 8.5cm width.
*b)* Scissors.

### Procedure
1 Position the patient in comfort with the affected arm exposed.
2 Cut a length of about 30cm of elasticated tubular support.
3 Position the support around the elbow, from one hand-span above to one hand-span below.
4 Turn back the edges to prevent fraying. (Figure **3**)
5 Ensure the circulation is satisfactory: check the radial pulse.

### Advice to patients
Keep the support dry when being worn.
Remove the support for washing arm, then re-apply; the support can be washed separately.
Remove the support at night.
Use the support for as long as required.
Exercise and/or elevate the arm as advised by the doctor.

---

## 3 Elasticated tubular support: (B) to the wrist

### Uses
1 Joint effusions and sprains.
2 Soft tissue injuries.
3 Following aspiration of a ganglion.
4 Following removal of Plaster of Paris.

### Equipment
*a)* Elasticated tubular support, 7cm width.
*b)* Scissors.

### Procedure
1 Position the patient in comfort with the affected arm exposed.
2 Cut a length of about 35cm of elasticated tubular support.
3 Cut a small hole about 6cm from one end for the thumb.
4 Position the support on the patient's forearm with his thumb through the hole and turn back the edges, leaving the elbow and the knuckles free.
(Figures **4, 5**)
5 Ensure the circulation is satisfactory: check the colour and warmth of the hand.

### Advice to patients
Keep the support dry when being worn.
Remove the support for washing arm, then re-apply; the support can be washed separately.
Remove the support at night.
Use the support for as long as required.
Exercise and/or elevate the arm as advised by the doctor.

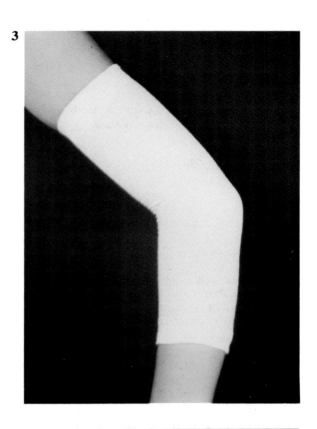

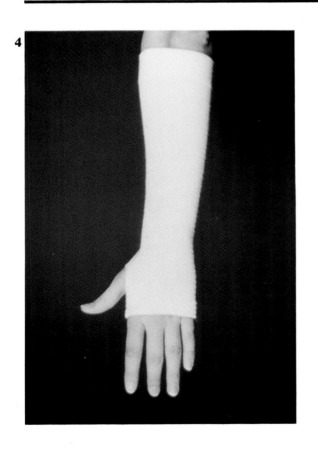

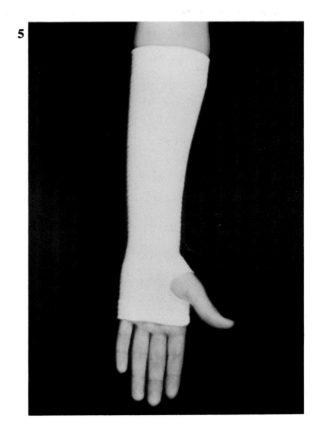

# 4 Elasticated tubular support: (C) to the knee

## Uses
1 Joint effusions and sprains.
2 Soft tissue injuries.
3 Following aspiration of the joint or a bursa.
4 Following removal of Plaster of Paris or Robert Jones pressure bandage.

## Equipment
*a)* Elasticated tubular support, 9.5cm width.
*b)* Applicator.
*c)* Scissors.

## Procedure
1 Position the patient in comfort with the affected leg exposed.
2 Cut a length of about 35cm of elasticated tubular support.
3 Thread the support on to the applicator.
4 Pass the applicator over the knee and position it a hand-span above the knee.
5 Remove the upper end of the support from the applicator and position it around the thigh. (Figure **6**)
6 Covering the knee with the support, slowly remove the applicator towards the foot.
7 Turn back the edges to prevent fraying. (Figure **7**)
8 Ensure the circulation is satisfactory: check the colour and warmth of the foot.

## Advice to patients
Keep the support dry when being worn.
Remove the support for washing leg, then re-apply; the support can be washed separately.
Remove the support at night.
Use the support for as long as required.
Exercise and/or elevate the leg as advised by the doctor.
A walking aid may be provided (see page 24).

---

# 5 Elasticated tubular support: (D) to the ankle

## Uses
1 Joint effusions and sprains.
2 Soft tissue injuries.
3 Following removal of Plaster of Paris.

## Equipment
*a)* Elasticated tubular support, 8.5cm width.
*b)* Applicator.
*c)* Scissors.

## Procedure
1 Position the patient in comfort with the affected leg exposed.
2 Cut a length of about 70cm of elasticated tubular support.
3 Thread the support on to the applicator.
4 Pass the applicator over the foot and position it 3cm below the knee.
5 Remove the upper end of the support from the applicator and position it around the limb. (Figure **8**)
6 Covering the lower leg, ankle and foot with the support, slowly remove the applicator towards the foot.
7 Turn back the edges to prevent fraying and ensure the knee and toes are free. (Figure **9**)
8 Ensure the circulation is satisfactory: check the colour and warmth of the foot.
*N.B.* For extra strength, cut a length of about 140cm and double back the support. (Figure **10**)

## Advice to patients
Keep the support dry when being worn.
Remove the support for washing leg, then re-apply; the support can be washed separately.
Remove the support at night.
Use the support for as long as required.
Exercise and/or elevate the leg as advised by the doctor.
A walking aid may be provided (see page 24).

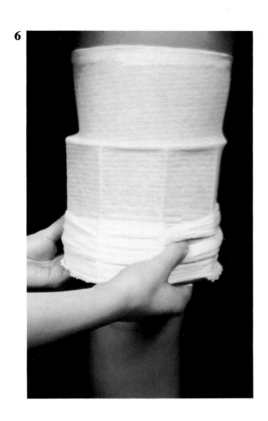

6

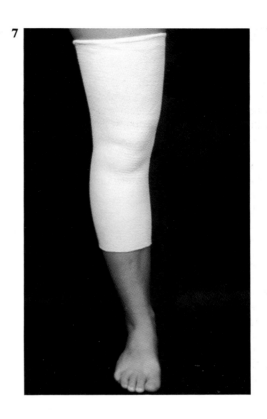

7

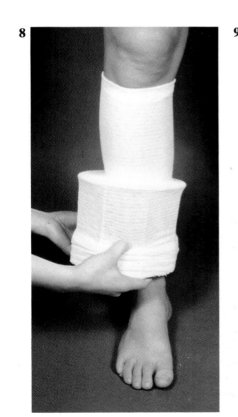

8

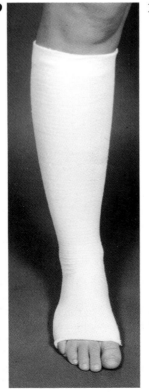

9

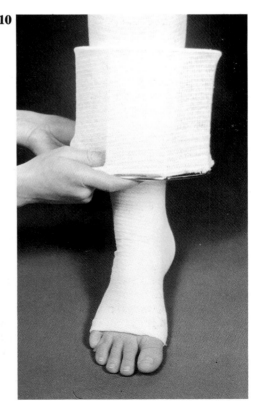

10

# 6 Crepe bandage: (A) to the elbow

## Uses
1 Support for sprains or bruises.
2 Following removal of Plaster of Paris.
3 As a pressure dressing, to reduce swelling or prevent bleeding.

## Equipment
a) Crepe bandage, 10cm width.
b) Elastic adhesive tape, 2.5cm width.
c) Scissors.

## Procedure
1 Position the patient in comfort with the affected arm exposed.
2 With the elbow slightly flexed, apply the bandage in a spiral fashion from one hand-span below the elbow to one hand-span above the elbow.
3 Secure with elastic adhesive tape. (Figure 11)

## Advice to patients
Keep the bandage dry when being worn.
Remove the bandage for washing, then re-apply.
Use the bandage for as long as advised.
Exercise and/or elevate the arm as advised by the doctor.

---

# 7 Crepe bandage: (B) to the wrist

## Uses
1 Support for sprains or bruises.
2 Following removal of Plaster of Paris.
3 As a pressure dressing, to reduce swelling or prevent bleeding.

## Equipment
a) Crepe bandage, 7.5cm width.
b) Elastic adhesive tape, 2.5cm width.
c) Scissors.

## Procedure
1 Position the patient in comfort with the affected arm exposed and the hand in a neutral position.
2 Anchor the bandage around the wrist with a fixing turn.
3 Proceed around the hand in a figure-of-eight fashion at least twice. (Figures 12, 13)
4 Continue up the forearm in a spiral fashion, covering two-thirds of the width of the bandage with each turn, to about 3cm below the elbow.
5 Secure with elastic adhesive tape.
6 Ensure the fingers and thumb are free for exercises. (Figure 14)

## Advice to patients
Keep the bandage dry when being worn.
Remove the bandage for washing, then re-apply.
Use the bandage for as long as advised.
Exercise and/or elevate the arm as advised by the doctor.

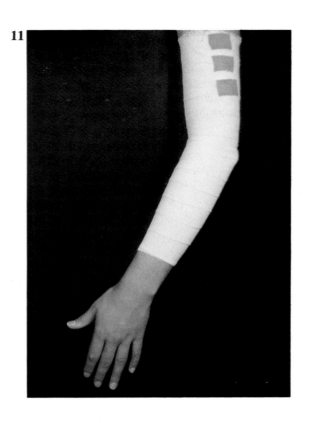

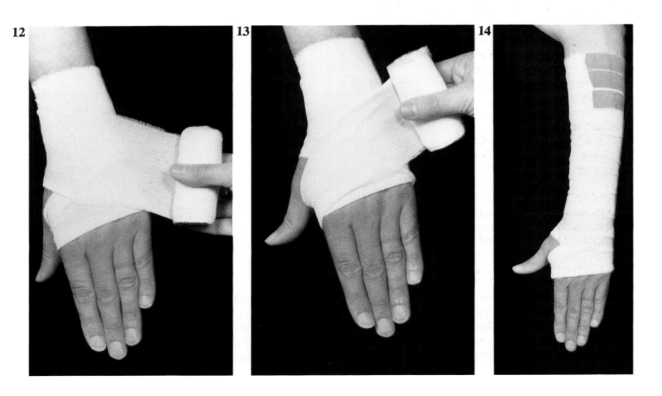

# 8  Crepe bandage: (C) to the knee

## Uses
1  Support for sprains or bruises.
2  Following removal of Plaster of Paris.
3  As a pressure dressing, to reduce swelling or prevent bleeding.

## Equipment
a)  2 crepe bandages, 15cm width.
b)  Elastic adhesive tape, 2.5cm width.
c)  Scissors.

## Procedure
1  Position the patient in comfort with the affected leg exposed.
2  Apply the first bandage in a spiral fashion from one hand-span below the knee joint to one hand-span above the knee joint.
3  Apply the second bandage in the reverse direction.
4  Secure with elastic adhesive tape. (Figures **15, 16**)

## Advice to patients
Keep the bandage dry when being worn.
Remove the bandage for washing, then re-apply.
Use the bandage for as long as advised.
Exercise and/or elevate the leg as advised by the doctor.

---

# 9  Crepe bandage: (D) to the ankle

## Uses
1  Support for sprains or bruises.
2  Following removal of Plaster of Paris.
3  As a pressure dressing, to reduce swelling or prevent bleeding.

## Equipment
a)  2 crepe bandages, 10cm width.
b)  Elastic adhesive tape, 2.5cm width.
c)  Scissors.

## Procedure
1  Position the patient in comfort with the affected leg exposed.
2  Position the foot at right angles to the leg.
3  Anchor the bandage around the foot with a fixing turn at the base of the toes.
4  Proceed around the foot in a spiral fashion until the ankle is reached.
5  Use two or three figure-of-eight turns around the ankle.
6  Continue up the leg in a spiral fashion, covering two-thirds of the width of the bandage with each turn, to about 3cm below the knee.
7  Ensure the toes are free.
8  Secure with elastic adhesive tape. (Figure **17**)

## Advice to patients
Keep the bandage dry when being worn.
Remove the bandage for washing, then re-apply.
Use the bandage for as long as advised.
Exercise and/or elevate the leg as advised by the doctor.

**15**

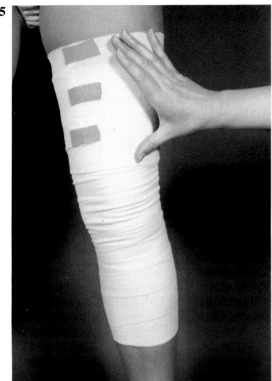

**16**

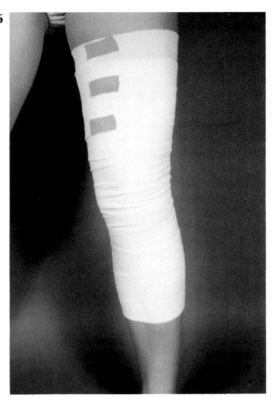

**17**

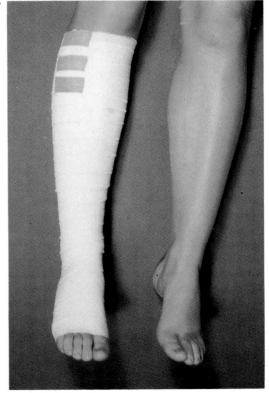

# 10 Wool and crepe bandage: (A) to the knee

## Uses
1 Injuries of the knee.
2 Effusions of the knee.
3 Following knee aspiration.

## Equipment
a) Cotton wool roll, 35cm width.
b) Crepe bandage, 15cm width.
c) Elastic adhesive tape, 2.5cm width.
d) Scissors.

## Procedure
1 Position the patient in comfort on a trolley, with the affected knee exposed and in about 10° of flexion.
2 Apply the cotton wool roll from one hand-span above the knee joint to one hand-span below the knee joint. (Figure **18**)
3 Cover the wool with crepe bandage in a spiral fashion.
4 Secure with elastic adhesive tape. (Figure **19**)

## Advice to patients
Keep the bandage dry when being worn.
Keeping the bandage on, exercise the ankle and quadriceps muscle as follows: hold the foot at right angles and tighten the muscle at the front of the thigh; raise the straightened leg for five seconds and lower it slowly; rotate the ankle clockwise and anti-clockwise. Repeat these exercises for five minutes every hour, during the day.
Elevate the leg when sitting or lying.
Use a walking aid according to the doctor's instructions (see page 24).

# 11 Wool and crepe bandage: (B) to the ankle

## Uses
1 Injuries of the ankle.
2 Swelling of the ankle.

## Equipment
a) Cotton wool roll, 35cm width.
b) 2 crepe bandages, 10cm width.
c) Elastic adhesive tape, 2.5cm width.
d) Scissors.

## Procedure
N.B. Two nurses are needed.
1 Position the patient in comfort, with the leg exposed from the knee downwards, and with the foot, supported by a nurse, at right angles to the leg.
2 Apply the cotton wool roll from the base of the toes to below the knee. (Figure **20**)
3 Cover the wool firmly with crepe bandage in a spiral fashion.
4 Secure with elastic adhesive tape. (Figure **21**)

## Advice to patients
Keep the bandage dry when being worn.
Move the knee and toes.
Elevate the leg as much as possible for the time advised by the doctor.
Use a walking aid according to the doctor's instructions (see page 24).

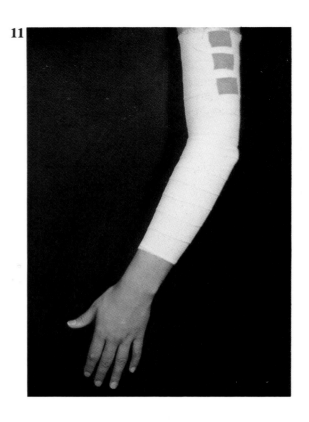

**11**

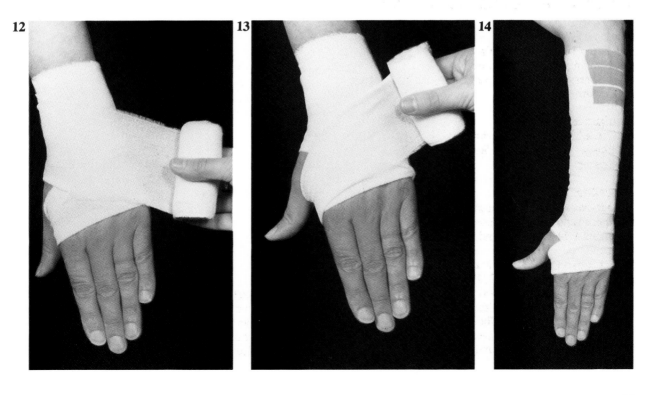

**12**

**13**

**14**

## 8 Crepe bandage: (C) to the knee

**Uses**
1 Support for sprains or bruises.
2 Following removal of Plaster of Paris.
3 As a pressure dressing, to reduce swelling or prevent bleeding.

**Equipment**
*a)* 2 crepe bandages, 15cm width.
*b)* Elastic adhesive tape, 2.5cm width.
*c)* Scissors.

**Procedure**
1 Position the patient in comfort with the affected leg exposed.
2 Apply the first bandage in a spiral fashion from one hand-span below the knee joint to one hand-span above the knee joint.
3 Apply the second bandage in the reverse direction.
4 Secure with elastic adhesive tape. (Figures **15, 16**)

**Advice to patients**
Keep the bandage dry when being worn.
Remove the bandage for washing, then re-apply.
Use the bandage for as long as advised.
Exercise and/or elevate the leg as advised by the doctor.

---

## 9 Crepe bandage: (D) to the ankle

**Uses**
1 Support for sprains or bruises.
2 Following removal of Plaster of Paris.
3 As a pressure dressing, to reduce swelling or prevent bleeding.

**Equipment**
*a)* 2 crepe bandages, 10cm width.
*b)* Elastic adhesive tape, 2.5cm width.
*c)* Scissors.

**Procedure**
1 Position the patient in comfort with the affected leg exposed.
2 Position the foot at right angles to the leg.
3 Anchor the bandage around the foot with a fixing turn at the base of the toes.
4 Proceed around the foot in a spiral fashion until the ankle is reached.
5 Use two or three figure-of-eight turns around the ankle.
6 Continue up the leg in a spiral fashion, covering two-thirds of the width of the bandage with each turn, to about 3cm below the knee.
7 Ensure the toes are free.
8 Secure with elastic adhesive tape. (Figure **17**)

**Advice to patients**
Keep the bandage dry when being worn.
Remove the bandage for washing, then re-apply.
Use the bandage for as long as advised.
Exercise and/or elevate the leg as advised by the doctor.

**15**

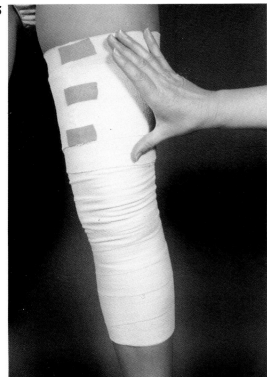

**16**

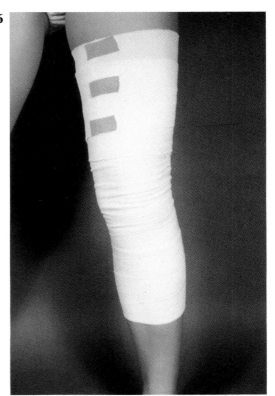

**17**

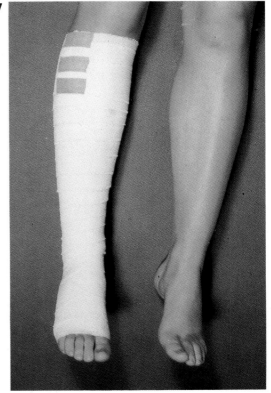

# 10 Wool and crepe bandage: (A) to the knee

## Uses
1 Injuries of the knee.
2 Effusions of the knee.
3 Following knee aspiration.

## Equipment
*a)* Cotton wool roll, 35cm width.
*b)* Crepe bandage, 15cm width.
*c)* Elastic adhesive tape, 2.5cm width.
*d)* Scissors.

## Procedure
1 Position the patient in comfort on a trolley, with the affected knee exposed and in about 10° of flexion.
2 Apply the cotton wool roll from one hand-span above the knee joint to one hand-span below the knee joint. (Figure **18**)
3 Cover the wool with crepe bandage in a spiral fashion.
4 Secure with elastic adhesive tape. (Figure **19**)

## Advice to patients
Keep the bandage dry when being worn.
Keeping the bandage on, exercise the ankle and quadriceps muscle as follows: hold the foot at right angles and tighten the muscle at the front of the thigh; raise the straightened leg for five seconds and lower it slowly; rotate the ankle clockwise and anti-clockwise. Repeat these exercises for five minutes every hour, during the day.
Elevate the leg when sitting or lying.
Use a walking aid according to the doctor's instructions (see page 24).

---

# 11 Wool and crepe bandage: (B) to the ankle

## Uses
1 Injuries of the ankle.
2 Swelling of the ankle.

## Equipment
*a)* Cotton wool roll, 35cm width.
*b)* 2 crepe bandages, 10cm width.
*c)* Elastic adhesive tape, 2.5cm width.
*d)* Scissors.

## Procedure
*N.B.* Two nurses are needed.
1 Position the patient in comfort, with the leg exposed from the knee downwards, and with the foot, supported by a nurse, at right angles to the leg.
2 Apply the cotton wool roll from the base of the toes to below the knee. (Figure **20**)
3 Cover the wool firmly with crepe bandage in a spiral fashion.
4 Secure with elastic adhesive tape. (Figure **21**)

## Advice to patients
Keep the bandage dry when being worn.
Move the knee and toes.
Elevate the leg as much as possible for the time advised by the doctor.
Use a walking aid according to the doctor's instructions (see page 24).

**18**

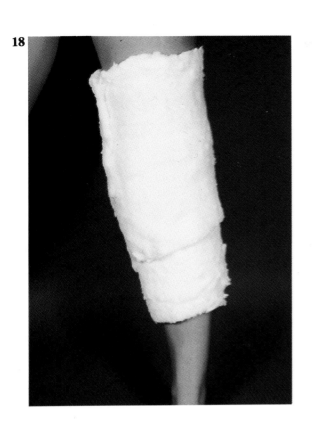

**19**

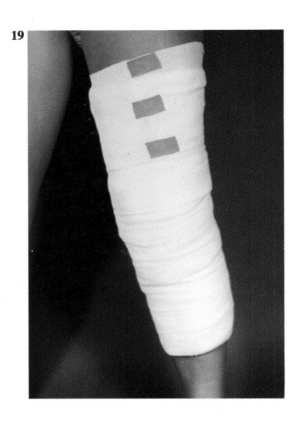

**20**

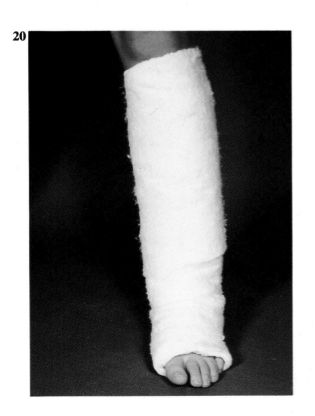

**21**

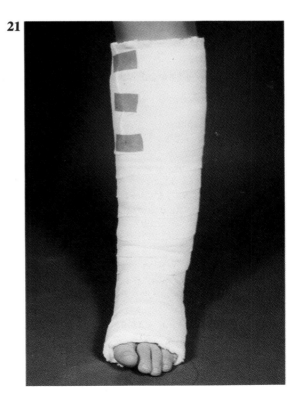

# 12 Neighbour strapping

## Uses
1 Fractures, sprains or bruises of the fingers or toes.
2 Following reduction of dislocated fingers or toes.

## Equipment
*a)* Cotton tubular bandage, 1.5cm width.
*b)* Elastic adhesive tape, 2.5cm width.
*c)* Scissors.

## Procedure
1 Position the patient in comfort with the affected fingers or toes exposed. Avoid strapping the index finger if possible, thus allowing the patient greater use of the hand.
2 Cut two lengths of cotton tubular bandage, each about 12cm long.
3 Put the cotton tubular bandage on to the two selected fingers and turn the cut edges over to prevent fraying.
4 Cut two lengths of elastic adhesive tape and apply one above and one below the proximal interphalangeal joint, strapping the two fingers together. (Figures **22, 23**)
5 Ensure that the circulation in the fingers is satisfactory (warm and pink) and the strapping is comfortable.

## Advice to patients
Keep the strapping dry.
Exercise the fingers within the limits of the strapping.
Do not remove the strapping until instructed to do so.

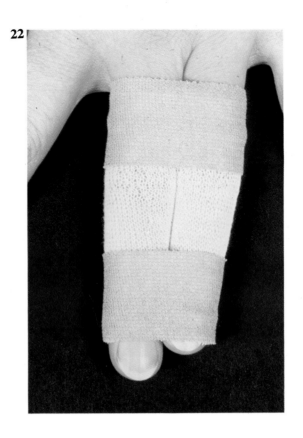

**22**

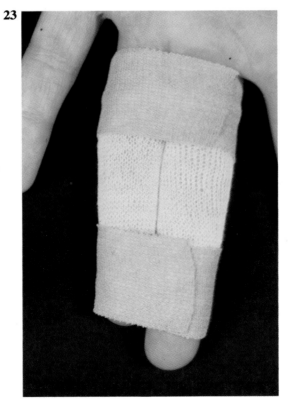

**23**

# 13 Zinc paste and ichthammol bandage

## Uses
1 Lacerations of thin and fragile skin.
2 Varicose eczema and leg ulcers.

## Equipment
*a)* Zinc paste and ichthammol bandage.
*b)* Cotton conforming bandage, 10cm width.
*c)* Elastic adhesive tape, 2.5cm width.
*d)* Gauze.
*e)* Scissors.

## Procedure
1 Wound toilet will have been performed already (see page 70). (Figures **24, 25**)
2 The zinc paste and ichthammol bandage is applied directly on to the wound in a continuous spiral, each turn overlapping the previous layer by two-thirds of its width. It is pleated and moulded as required to accommodate the contours of the limb. (Figures **26, 27**)
3 For the lower limb, the foot is positioned at right angles to the leg and the bandage is applied from the base of the toes to just below the knee.
4 If there is likely to be excessive exudate from the wound, gauze may be applied on top of the zinc paste and ichthammol bandage, over the wound. (Figure **28**)
5 The entire dressing is covered with cotton conforming bandage, secured with elastic adhesive tape. (Figure **29**)

## Advice to patients
Keep the dressing dry.
Keep the limb elevated as much as possible.

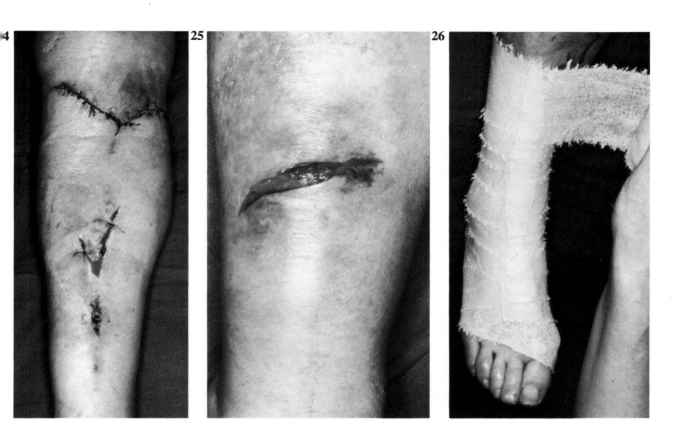

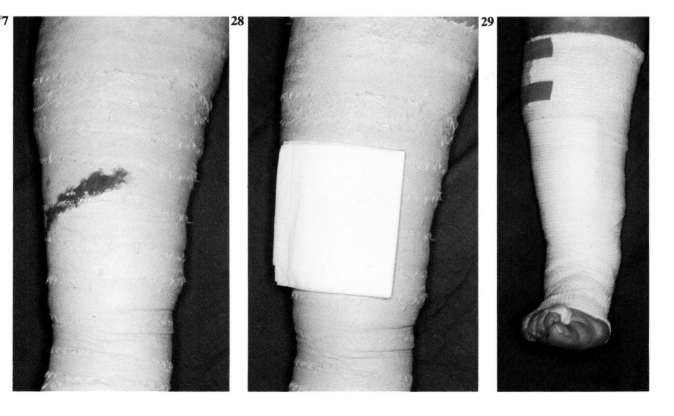

# 14 Walking aids

## WALKING-STICKS

With the patient standing straight, arms by the sides, measure from the wrists to the floor: this is the correct length for the stick.

Ensure that the rubber on the stick has enough tread.

The stick must always be placed on firm dry ground. Flat shoes should be worn.

When walking, the stick is held in the hand opposite to the injured leg. It is held in front of the patient and a little to the side (Figure **30**). The stick is put forward first, followed by a small step with the injured leg, followed by a bigger step with the uninjured leg.

Short steps are used for turning.

When going upstairs, the stick is held on the side of the injured leg. The first step is taken with the uninjured leg*; then the injured leg and stick are brought up to the same step.

When going downstairs, the stick is held on the side of the injured leg. The first step is taken with the injured leg* and stick together; then the uninjured leg is taken down to the same step.

*'Good leg *up* first. Bad leg *down* first.'

## CRUTCHES

With the patient standing straight, measure from the axilla to the floor: the crutches should be 5cm shorter than this length.

Ensure that the rubbers on the crutches have enough tread and all nuts are tightened.

The crutches must always be placed on firm dry ground. Flat shoes should be worn.

The patient's weight is borne by his hands on the handgrips and not by his axillae. The elbows should be slightly flexed (Figure **31**). One crutch should be placed under each axilla and the handgrips held firmly. The patient squeezes his upper arms towards his body to hold the crutches firmly. He bears weight on one foot, places the crutches on the floor 30cm in front of his feet and swings his body forwards through the crutches.

The patient moves upstairs or downstairs on his bottom.

To sit down, the patient removes the crutches from his axillae and holds them in one hand, using the other hand to steady the chair.

## FRAMES

With the patient standing straight, arms by the sides, measure from the wrists to the floor: select a frame as near as possible to this height.

Ensure that the rubbers on the frame have enough tread.

All four legs of the frame must always be placed firmly on dry ground. Flat shoes should be worn.

The patient stands with the frame in front of him and leans forwards on to the frame, holding the handgrips firmly. (Figure **32**)

For partial weight-bearing, the frame is moved slightly forwards, then the injured leg is brought forwards, then the uninjured leg is brought slightly past the injured leg. The arms take the weight of the body. The patient must not step too far forwards into the frame or he may overbalance.

For non-weight-bearing, the frame is moved slightly forwards and the patient then hops forwards. The patient must not step too far forwards into the frame or he may overbalance.

Short steps are used for turning; the frame is moved, then the injured leg, then the uninjured leg.

The patient moves upstairs or downstairs on his bottom.

**30**

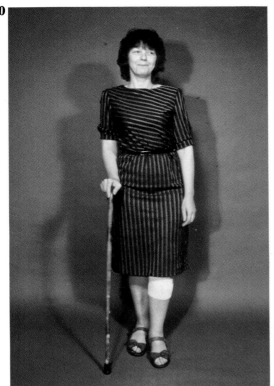

**31**

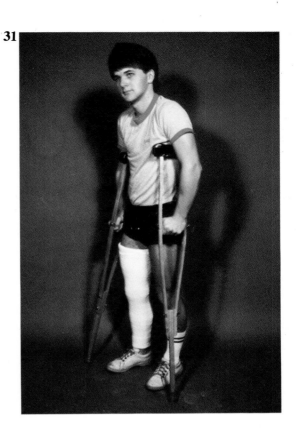

**32**

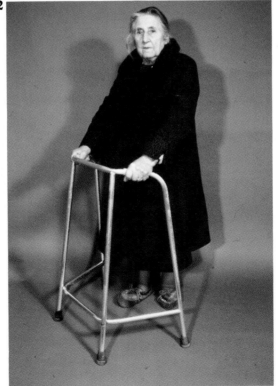

# 15 Collar and cuff

## Uses
1 Fracture of the clavicle.
2 Fracture of the neck, shaft or supracondylar region of the humerus.
3 Following reduction of a dislocated shoulder or a dislocated elbow.
4 Infections of the elbow; olecranon bursitis.
5 To support an above-elbow Plaster of Paris cast.

## Equipment
*a)* Collar and cuff: different types are available.
*b)* Elastic adhesive tape, 2.5cm width.
*c)* Axillary pad (optional).
*d)* Scissors.
*e)* Talcum powder.
*f)* Towel.
*g)* Soap and water.

## Procedure
1 Undress the patient to the waist and remove all jewellery.
2 Wash, dry and powder the axilla.
3 Position the affected arm so that the elbow is at a right angle or higher.
4 Tie the small piece of leather around the wrist, tightly enough to prevent removal of the hand. (Figure **33**) (If the collar and cuff is to be worn over the clothes, tie the wrist piece more loosely to allow removal of the hand.)
5 Place the large piece of leather around the neck, with the stitched side uppermost to prevent irritation.
6 Tie both loose ends of bandage together. (Figure **34**)
7 Cut off the loose ends.
8 Secure the knot with elastic adhesive tape. (Figures **35, 36**)
9 An axillary pad may be used between the upper arm and the chest wall to prevent chafing. (Figures **37, 38**)
10 For children, it is advisable to continue the elastic adhesive tape from the wrist to the neck to prevent removal of the collar over the head.
11 Check the radial pulse and the colour and sensation of the fingers.

## Advice to patients
Exercise the uninjured joints of the arm, according to the doctor's instructions.
If the arm becomes discoloured or numb, return to hospital.
Apply powder at the neck and wrist to prevent chafing.
Wear the collar and cuff continuously, day and night (unless the doctor instructs otherwise).
An old tee-shirt or vest, split at one shoulder, may be worn to prevent the arm rubbing against the chest wall.

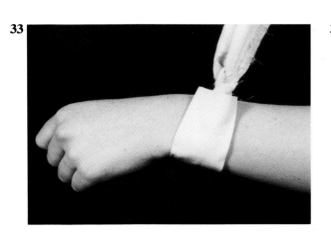

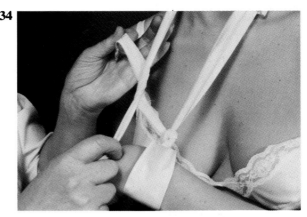

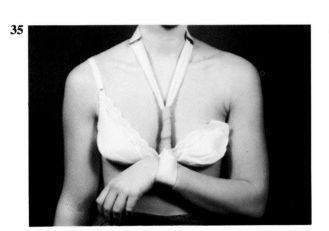

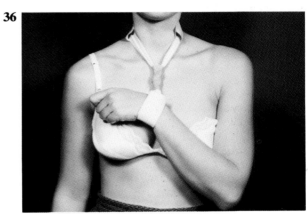

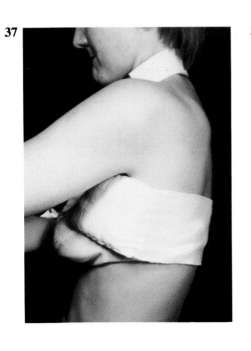

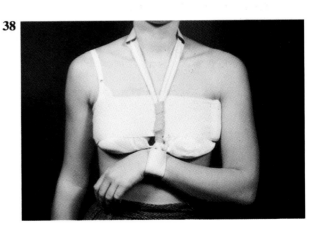

# 16 Broad arm sling

## Uses
1 Fractures of the clavicle, humerus, elbow, forearm, wrist or metacarpals.
2 Following reduction of a dislocated shoulder, dislocated elbow or dislocated fingers.
3 Infected wounds of the hand or forearm.
4 To support an above-elbow Plaster of Paris cast or any injured arm.

## Equipment
a) Sling.
b) Safety pin (for an adult).
c) Elastic adhesive tape, 2.5cm width (for a child).
d) Scissors.

## Procedure
1 Undress the patient to the waist if the sling is to be worn under the clothes. Remove all jewellery.
2 Position the patient in comfort with the elbow at right angles.
3 Place the long straight side of the sling in line with the sternum and place the apex of the sling behind the injured arm. Extend the upper end of the sling over the opposite shoulder. (Figure **39**)
4 Bring the lower end of the sling over the shoulder of the injured arm. Tie the two ends behind the neck.
5 Secure the elbow in the sling with a safety pin (or elastic adhesive tape for a child). (Figure **40**)

## Advice to patients
Exercise the uninjured joints, according to the doctor's instructions.

Follow the doctor's instructions as to whether or not the sling is to be worn at night. If it is to be removed at night, a relative should be shown how to re-apply the sling.

The sling should be worn for as long as the doctor advises.

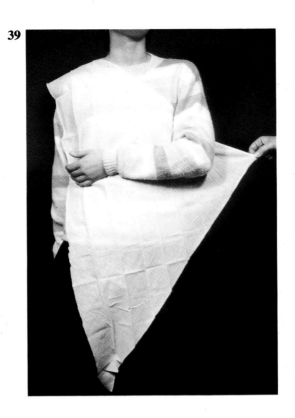

**39**

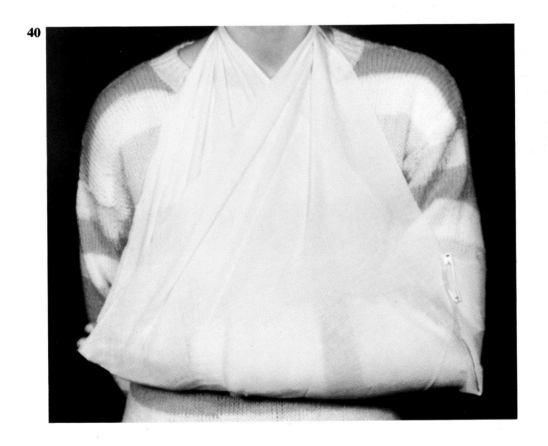

**40**

# 17 High sling

## Uses
1 The same as for a Broad Arm Sling (see page 28).
2 To arrest haemorrhage (with a pressure dressing).
3 To reduce swelling of the forearm, wrist or hand.

## Equipment
*a)* Sling.
*b)* Two safety pins (for an adult).
*c)* One self-locking safety pin (for a child).
*d)* Elastic adhesive tape, 2.5cm width (for a child).
*e)* Scissors.

## Procedure
1 Undress the patient to the waist if the sling is to be worn under the clothes. Remove all jewellery.
2 Position the patient in comfort.
3 Place the long straight side of the sling in line with the sternum and place the apex of the sling behind the injured arm. Extend the upper end of the sling over the opposite shoulder. (Figure **41**)
4 Bring the lower end of the sling over the shoulder of the injured arm. Tie the two ends behind the neck.
5 Secure the elbow in the sling with a safety pin (or elastic adhesive tape for a child). (Figure **42**)
6 Raise the hand of the injured arm up to the opposite shoulder and tighten the sling with a safety pin (self-locking type for a child). (Figure **43**)

## Advice to patients
Exercise the uninjured joints according to the doctor's instructions.
Remove the sling at night but try to sleep with the affected arm resting up on two pillows. Instruct a relative how to re-apply the sling.
The sling should be worn for as long as the doctor advises.

**41**

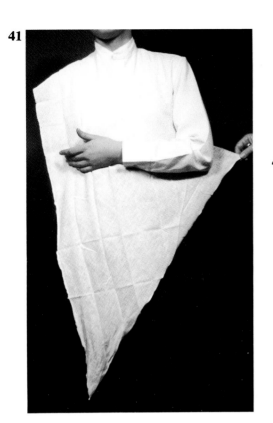

**42**

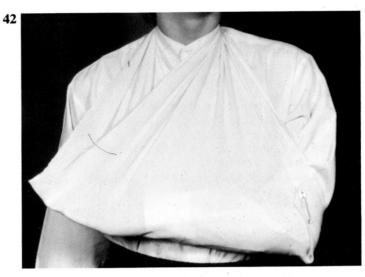

**43**

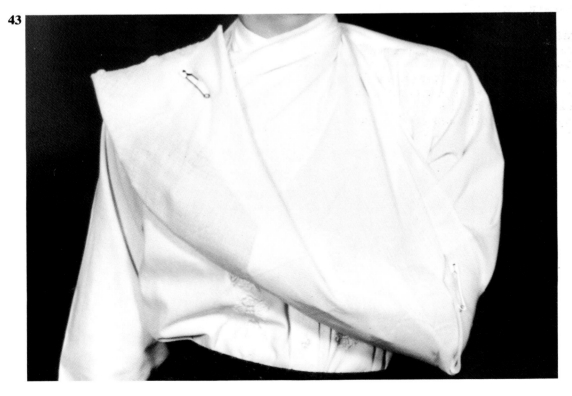

# 18 Wrist strapping

## Uses
1 Sprains, bruises or minor fractures of the wrist.
2 Following removal of Plaster of Paris.

## Equipment
*a)* Cotton tubular bandage, 5cm width.
*b)* Elastic adhesive tape, 5cm width.
*c)* Scissors.

## Procedure
1 Expose the affected arm from the elbow downwards. Remove all jewellery from the limb. Place the hand in the neutral position.
2 Check that the patient is not allergic to elastic adhesive tape; if so, substitute a non-allergenic tape.
3 When using elastic adhesive tape, allow its natural tension to be released as it is unrolled, to avoid constriction of the arm.
4 Cut a piece of cotton tubular bandage about 40cm long.
5 Cut a small hole about 6cm from one end for the thumb.
6 Apply the bandage to the arm from the knuckles to the elbow, with the thumb through the hole, and turn back the ends.
7 Unroll the elastic adhesive tape. Anchor the tape around the wrist with a fixing turn and proceed around the hand in a figure-of-eight fashion at least twice, snipping the tape to accommodate the thumb. Continue over the wrist and forearm in a spiral fashion, covering half the width of the tape with each turn. Anchor the tape to the skin about 3cm below the elbow. (Figures **44, 45**)

## Advice to patients
Keep the strapping dry.
If the fingers become discoloured or numb, return to hospital.
Exercise the uninjured joints according to the doctor's instructions.
Elevate the arm in a sling if advised by the doctor.
The strapping is usually left in place for 7 to 10 days; after this time remove it, following the doctor's instructions.

**44**

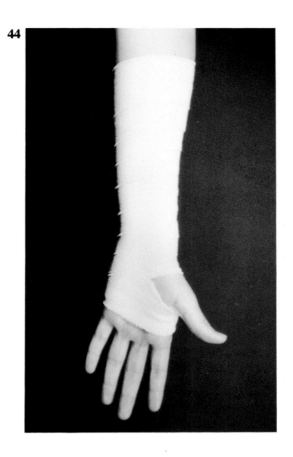

**45**

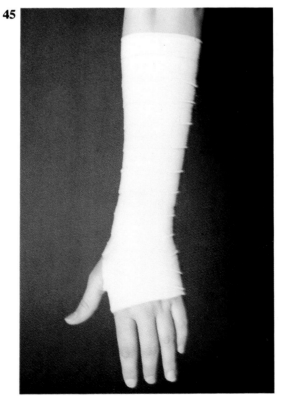

# 19 Metacarpal pad and strapping

## Use
Support of metacarpal fractures.

## Equipment
a) Cotton tubular bandage, 5cm width.
b) Elastic adhesive tape, 5cm width.
c) Adhesive orthopaedic felt, 5-10mm thickness (depending on the patient's size, injury and occupation).
d) Scissors.

## Procedure
1 Expose the affected arm from the elbow downwards. Remove all jewellery from the arm.
2 Check that the patient is not allergic to elastic adhesive tape; if so, substitute a non-allergenic tape.
3 Cut a piece of cotton tubular bandage about 40cm long.
4 Cut a small hole about 6cm from one end for the thumb.
5 Apply the bandage to the forearm from the knuckles to the elbow, with the thumb through the hole, and turn back the ends.
6 Measure and cut a piece of orthopaedic felt to fit into the palm of the hand and cut out an arc to allow movement of the thumb.
7 Stick the felt on to the bandage on the palm. (Figure **46**)
8 Unroll the elastic adhesive tape. Anchor the tape around the wrist with a fixing turn and proceed around the hand in a figure-of-eight fashion at least twice, snipping the tape to accommodate the thumb. Continue over the wrist and forearm in a spiral fashion, covering half the width of the tape with each turn. Anchor the tape to the skin about 3cm below the elbow. (Figures **47, 48**)

## Advice to patients
Keep the strapping dry.
If the fingers become discoloured or numb, return to hospital.
Exercise the uninjured joints according to the doctor's instructions.
Elevate the arm in a sling if advised by the doctor.

**46**

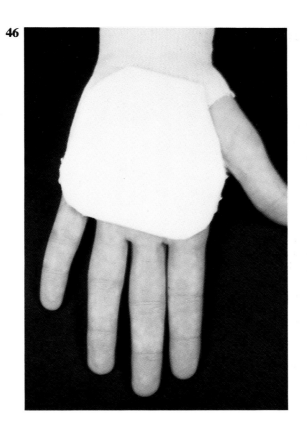

**47**

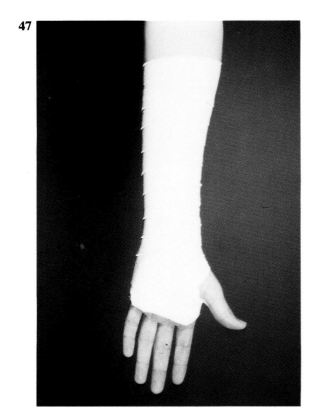

**48**

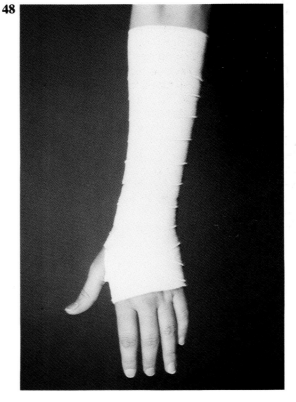

# 20 Strapping over roller bandage

## Use
Fractures of the fingers or metacarpal heads.

## Equipment
a) Cotton conforming bandage, 5cm width.
b) Cotton tubular bandage, 1.5cm width.
c) Crepe bandage, 7.5cm width.
d) Elastic adhesive tape, 2.5cm width.
e) Scissors.
f) Razor.

## Procedure
1 Check that the patient is not allergic to elastic adhesive tape: if so, substitute a non-allergenic tape.
2 Expose the affected arm from the elbow downwards. Remove all jewellery from the limb. Shave the back of the hand to the wrist if necessary.
3 Apply a 10cm length of cotton tubular bandage to the injured finger and a 10cm length to one (or two) of the neighbouring fingers. Fold back the cut edges to prevent fraying. Avoid using the index finger if possible, thus allowing the patient greater use of the hand.
4 Place an unwound roll of cotton conforming bandage into the palm of the hand under the bandaged fingers.
5 Apply elastic adhesive tape from the dorsum of the wrist, along the line of the metacarpal, over the length of the bandaged finger and so to the palmar side of the wrist; apply traction as you do this, to position the fingers correctly. Repeat for the other bandaged finger(s).
6 Apply elastic adhesive tape around the wrist to secure the ends of the strips of tape which are already applied: leave a 2cm gap to avoid constriction. (Figures **49, 50**)
7 Cover the whole strapping with a crepe bandage and secure it with elastic adhesive tape, leaving the unbandaged finger(s) and the thumb free. (Figures **51, 52**)

## Advice to patients
Keep the strapping dry.
If the fingers become numb or severe pain or tingling develop, return to hospital.
Exercise the free fingers and thumb.
Elevate the arm in a sling if advised by the doctor.

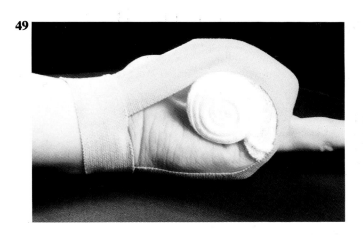

**49**

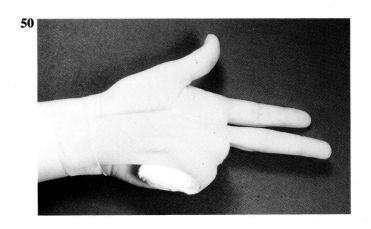

**50**

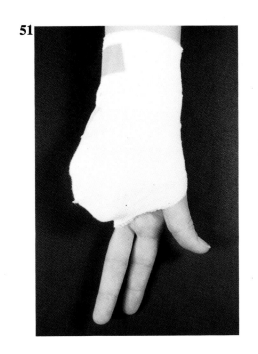

**51**

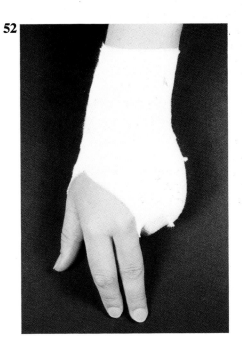

**52**

# 21 Thumb spica

## Uses
1 Fractures, sprains or bruises of the thumb.
2 Following reduction of a dislocated thumb.

## Equipment
*a)* Cotton tubular bandage, 1.5cm width.
*b)* Elastic adhesive tape, 2.5cm width.
*c)* Scissors.

## Procedure
1 Check that the patient is not allergic to elastic
   adhesive tape: if so, substitute a non-allergenic tape.
2 Cut a length of about 10cm of cotton tubular
   bandage, position it over the thumb and fold back the
   cut edges, leaving the tip of the thumb free.
3 Cut about eight pieces of elastic adhesive tape of
   varying lengths from 8cm to 15cm.
4 Apply the lengths of elastic adhesive tape from the tip
   of the thumb to the base in a figure-of-eight fashion,
   forming a 'V' from the nail to the base of the first
   metacarpal. Snip the tape as required. (Figure **53**)
5 Apply a length of elastic adhesive tape around the
   wrist to anchor the ends of the tape: leave a 2cm gap
   to avoid constriction. (Figures **54-56**)
6 Check the colour and sensation of the thumb.

## Advice to patients
Keep the spica dry.
If the thumb becomes discoloured or numb or severe
pain or tingling develop, return to hospital.
Wear the spica for as long as the doctor advises.

**53**

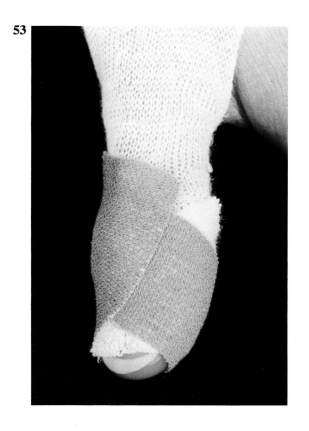

**54**

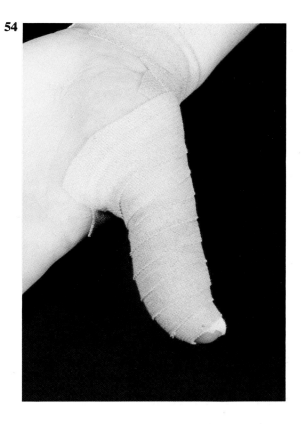

**55**

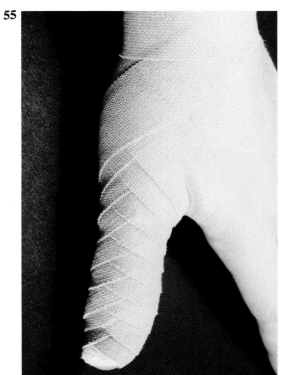

**56**

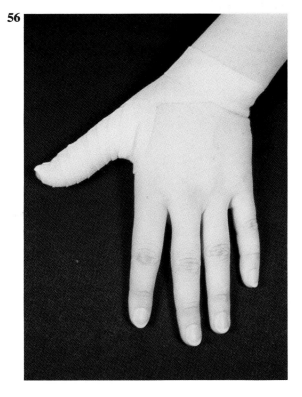

# 22 Mallet splint

## Use
Mallet finger, which is due to rupture of the terminal extensor tendon or avulsion of a fragment of its bony insertion.

## Equipment
*a)* Mallet finger splint, of the correct size; various types are in use.
*b)* Adhesive felt, 5mm thickness.
*c)* Elastic adhesive tape, 2.5cm width.
*d)* Scissors.

## Procedure
1 Check that the patient is not allergic to elastic adhesive tape: if so, substitute a non-allergenic tape.
2 Expose the affected finger; remove any rings; wash and dry the finger. (Figure **57***)*
3 Apply the splint to the finger, ensuring that the terminal joint is straight and neither flexed nor hyperextended. The end of the splint can be padded with felt if necessary (Figures **58, 59**). Ensure that the proximal joint is not splinted.
4 Attach the splint to the finger with elastic adhesive tape. (Figure **60**)

## Advice to patients
The splint must not be removed (except for reduced circulation) until the doctor so instructs.
Keep the finger as clean and dry as possible: a finger-stall is useful.
If the finger becomes discoloured or numb or severe pain or tingling develop, return to hospital.
Exercise the other joints of the hand, including the proximal joint of the affected finger.

**57**

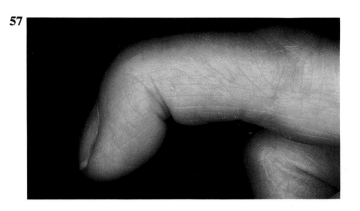

**58**

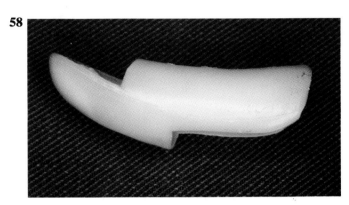

**59**

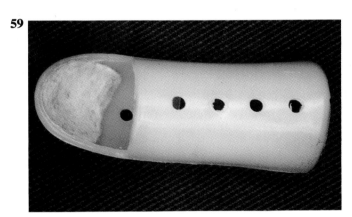

**60**

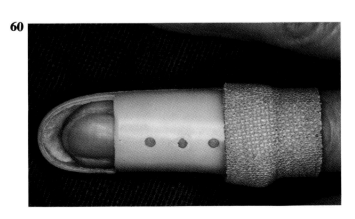

# 23 Application of skin extensions

## Use
To provide traction, either fixed or balanced, for the limb, indirectly through the skin:
1. fractured neck of femur.
2. fractured shaft of femur (prior to the application of Thomas' splint) (see page 44).
3. fractured tibial plateau.
4. fractured pelvis (especially central dislocation of the hip).
5. irritable hip.
6. low back pain.

## Equipment
a) Two rolls of elastic adhesive tape skin extensions, 7.5cm width, with attached webbing. Alternative types are available.
b) Two cotton conforming bandages, 10cm width.
c) Razor.
d) Tincture of benzoin spray.
e) White lint, 10cm width.
f) Needle.
g) Cotton.
h) Scissors.

## Procedure
*N.B.* Two nurses are needed.
Suitable analgesia is required, as prescribed by the doctor.

1. Check that the patient is not allergic to elastic adhesive tape: if so, latex foam rubber skin traction bandage can be substituted (this is used on patients with thin and fragile skin).
2. When using elastic adhesive tape, allow its natural tension to be released as it is unrolled.
3. Reassure the patient and explain the procedure.
4. Position the patient in comfort in a recumbent or semi-recumbent position on a trolley.
5. Expose the affected limb.
6. Shave the leg from the hip to the ankle on both the inside and outside of the limb.
7. Spray along both shaved areas with tincture of benzoin; this improves the adhesion of the skin extensions.
8. White lint, long enough to encircle the ankle, is folded double and sewn loosely around the malleoli to protect the bony prominences from friction.
9. Unroll the elastic adhesive tape skin extensions to the approximate length of the limb.
10. A nurse supports the patient's foot and raises the leg about 25cm from the trolley.
11. A second nurse applies the skin extension on the outside of the leg from above the lateral malleolus up to the greater trochanter.
12. The inside skin extension is then applied from the medial malleolus up to 5cm below the groin. (Figure **61**)
13. The extensions should be stretched sideways as they are applied upwards, thus accommodating the contours of the limb and preventing wrinkling. It may be necessary to snip the extensions at the knee joint to accommodate the contours. (Figure **62**)
14. Cotton conforming bandages are applied over the extensions, one above and one below the knee.
15. The conforming bandages are sewn into position. (Figure **63**)
16. The knee is left exposed to allow for physiotherapy, observation and different methods of traction.
17. The webbing is secured to the end of the trolley, thus aiding splintage, immobility and reduction of pain during transportation to the ward.
18. The patient is made comfortable and transported to the ward.

**61**

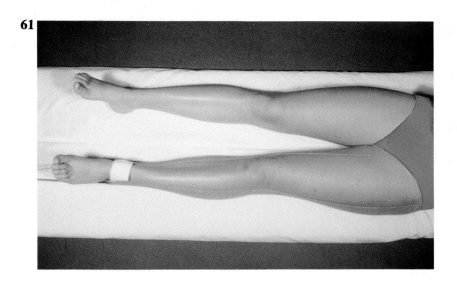

**62**

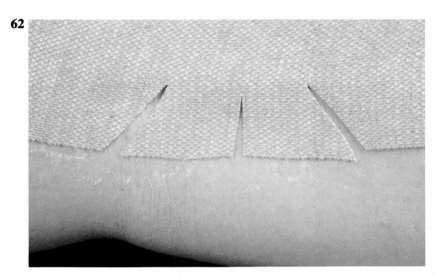

**63**

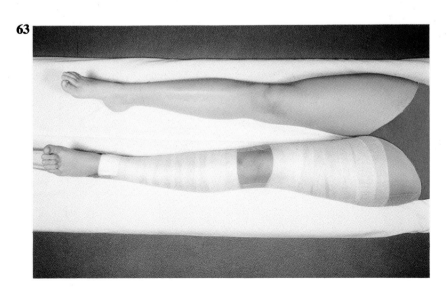

# 24 Thomas' splint

## Use
To provide support and/or splintage to the lower limb after injury (particularly fracture of the shaft of the femur) and provide fixed traction if required.

## Equipment
a) Thomas' splint.
b) Flannel bandage, 15cm width.
c) Roll of Gamgee dressing.
d) Two calico bandages, 15cm width.
e) Tape measure.
f) Safety nappy pins.
g) Scissors.
h) Needle.
i) Cotton.
j) Block.

## Procedure
N.B. One doctor and three nurses are needed.
Suitable analgesia is required, as prescribed by the doctor.

1 Explain the procedure to the patient. Skin extensions will have been applied already (see page 42).

2 Position the patient in a recumbent or semi-recumbent position, leaving the injured leg exposed.

3 Select the ring size of the splint by measuring around the thigh of the uninjured leg at the level of the groin and add 5cm to allow for swelling. Select the length of the splint by measuring the inside of the leg from the groin to the heel and add 25cm, as the splint must be long enough to permit full plantar flexion of the foot.

4 The doctor applies traction to the extension webbing and the splint is passed over the foot and positioned comfortably at the groin.

5 A nurse supports the fracture site during application of the splint.

6 A second nurse cuts the flannel bandage into about six lengths of approximately 60-90cm each, according to the size of the splint.

7 A nurse stands on each side of the trolley in order to apply the flannel to the splint, working from the top of the splint down to just above the patient's heel.

8 The second nurse threads the flannel around the inner metal bar and passes both ends under the leg. A third nurse collects the two ends and passes them over the outer bar, under the leg and back to the second nurse, who applies cross-traction by ensuring the flannel slings are taut. The third nurse applies two safety pins to each sling, underneath the splint just behind the outer bar. (Figure **64**)

9 Line the whole length of the splint with a piece of Gamgee. A pad of Gamgee is positioned under the knee. (Figure **65**)

10 The doctor attaches the extension webbings to the end of the Thomas' splint and ties them securely.

11 The end of the splint is supported on a block.

12 Calico bandages are applied over the splint, incorporating the slings of flannel: one is applied from ankle to knee and the other from above the knee to the ring of the splint. These are sewn into position with cotton. The knee is left free for observation and physiotherapy. (Figure **66**)

13 The patient is made comfortable and transported to the ward.

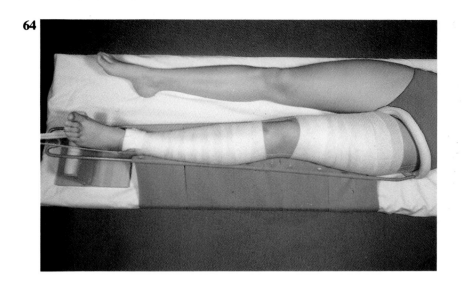

**64**

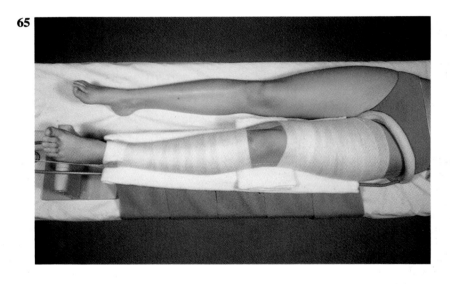

**65**

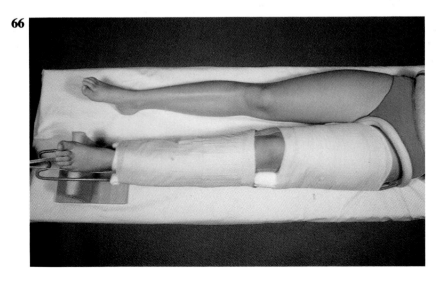

**66**

# 25 Robert Jones pressure bandage

## Uses
1 Effusion or haemarthrosis of the knee.
2 Following knee aspiration.
3 Following manipulation of a locked knee.

## Equipment
*a)* Cotton wool roll, 35cm width.
*b)* Three calico bandages, 15cm width.
*c)* Two crepe bandages, 15cm width.
*d)* Elastic adhesive tape, 2.5cm width.
*e)* Needle.
*f)* Cotton.
*g)* Scissors.

## Procedure
*N.B.* Two nurses are needed.
1 Position the patient in comfort on a trolley and remove all clothing from the affected leg.
2 A nurse holds the leg by the heel, ensuring that the knee is straight.
3 A second nurse applies a layer of cotton wool from above the malleoli to the top of the thigh. (Figure **67**)
4 Calico bandage is applied firmly to cover the cotton wool from above the malleoli to the thigh; it is sewn into position at the upper end. (Figure **68**)
5 A second layer of cotton wool is applied, followed by a second layer of calico bandage from the thigh to the ankle (i.e. in the reverse direction); it is sewn into position at the lower end.
6 A third layer of cotton wool and of calico can be applied, at the doctor's discretion.
7 Apply crepe bandages over the whole dressing and secure with elastic adhesive tape. (Figure **69**)

## Advice to patients
Keep the pressure bandage dry.
If the foot becomes discoloured, numb or excessively swollen, return to hospital.
Keeping the bandage on, exercise the ankle and quadriceps muscle as follows:
hold the foot at right angles and tighten the muscle at the front of the thigh; raise the straightened leg for five seconds and lower it slowly; rotate the ankle clockwise and anti-clockwise; repeat these exercises for five minutes every hour, during the day.
Elevate the limb according to the doctor's instructions.
Follow the doctor's advice regarding weight-bearing, mobility and walking aids (see page 24).
Do not remove the pressure bandage. The outer layer of crepe bandages may be removed for washing or neatening and re-applied.

**67**

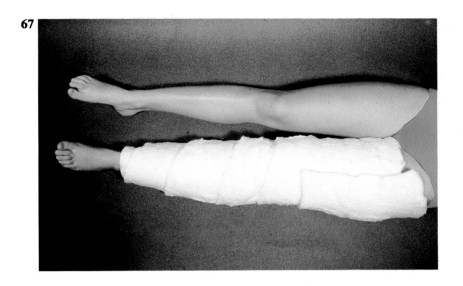

**68**

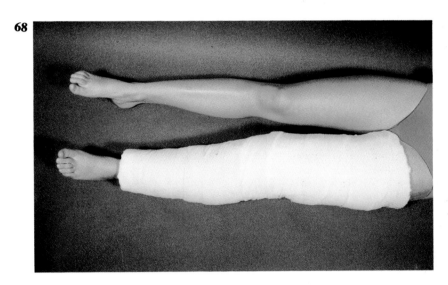

**69**

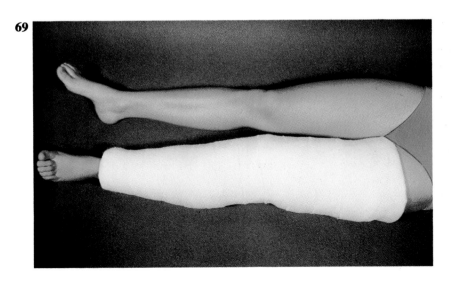

# 26 Ankle strapping

## Uses
1 Sprains of the ankle.
2 Minor fractures around the ankle.
3 Following removal of Plaster of Paris.

## Equipment
*a)* Cotton tubular bandage, 7.5cm width.
*b)* Two rolls of elastic adhesive tape, 7.5cm width.
*c)* Scissors.

## Procedure
1 Check that the patient is not allergic to elastic adhesive tape: if so, substitute a non-allergenic tape.
2 When using elastic adhesive tape, allow its natural tension to be released as it is unrolled, to avoid constriction of the limb.
3 Expose the affected leg from the knee downwards; position the foot at right angles to the leg.
4 Cut a piece of cotton tubular bandage about 70cm long. Apply this to the leg from the base of the toes to below the knee. Turn back the ends.
5 Unroll the elastic adhesive tape. Anchor the tape to the skin at the base of the toes, and work up the foot in a spiral fashion. Two or three figure-of-eight turns are applied around the ankle (Figure **70**). Ensure that all the cotton tubular bandage is covered at the heel. Continue up the leg in a spiral fashion, covering half of the width of the tape with each turn, and ensuring that the tape is free of creases, as these may cause a pressure sore. Anchor the tape to the skin about 3cm below the knee. (Figure **71**)

## Advice to patients
Keep the strapping dry.
If the toes become discoloured, numb or excessively swollen, return to hospital.
Exercise the toes by wriggling.
Elevate the foot above waist level as much as possible, particularly during the first 48 hours; rest the foot on two pillows at night.
Follow the doctor's advice regarding weight-bearing, mobility and walking aids (see page 24).
Remove the strapping according to the doctor's instructions.

**70**

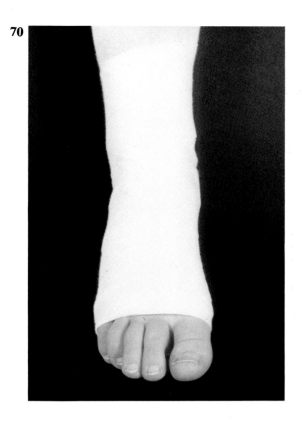

**71**

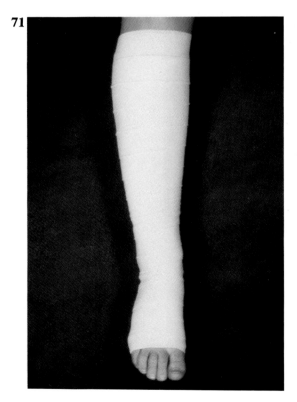

# 27 Metatarsal pad and strapping

## Uses
1 Fractures of the metatarsal bones.
2 Painful conditions of the foot.

## Equipment
*a)* Cotton tubular bandage, 7.5cm width.
*b)* Two rolls of elastic adhesive tape, 7.5cm width.
*c)* Adhesive orthopaedic felt, 5-10mm thickness.
*d)* Scissors.

## Procedure
1 Check that the patient is not allergic to elastic adhesive tape: if so, substitute a non-allergenic tape.
2 When using elastic adhesive tape, allow its natural tension to be released as it is unrolled, to avoid constriction of the limb.
3 Expose the affected leg from the knee downwards; position the foot at right angles to the leg.
4 Cut a piece of cotton tubular bandage about 70cm long. Apply this to the leg from the base of the toes to below the knee. Turn back the ends.
5 Measure and cut a pad of orthopaedic felt and apply it to the cotton tubular bandage under the painful area. (Figure **72**)
6 Unroll the elastic adhesive tape. Anchor the tape to the skin at the base of the toes, and work up the foot in a spiral fashion. Two or three figure-of-eight turns are applied around the ankle. Ensure that all the cotton tubular bandage is covered at the heel. Continue up the leg in a spiral fashion, covering half of the width of the tape with each turn, and ensuring that the tape is free of creases, as these may cause a pressure sore. Anchor the tape to the skin about 3cm below the knee. (Figures **73, 74**)

## Advice to patients
Keep the strapping dry.
If the toes become discoloured, numb or excessively swollen, return to hospital.
Exercise the toes by wriggling.
Elevate the foot above waist level as much as possible, particularly during the first 48 hours; rest the foot on two pillows at night.
Follow the doctor's advice regarding weight-bearing, mobility and walking aids (see page 24).
Remove the strapping according to the doctor's instructions.

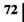**72**

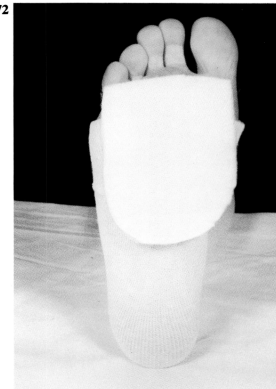

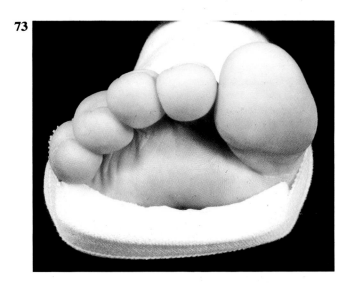**73**

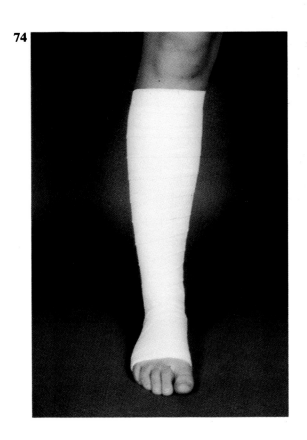**74**

# 28 Toe spica

## Uses
1 Fractures, sprains or bruises of the great toe.
2 Following reduction of a dislocated great toe.

## Equipment
*a)* Cotton tubular bandage, 2.5cm width.
*b)* Elastic adhesive tape, 2.5cm width.
*c)* Scissors.

## Procedure
1 Check that the patient is not allergic to elastic adhesive tape: if so, substitute a non-allergenic tape.
2 Cut a length of about 8cm of cotton tubular bandage, position it over the toe and fold back the cut edges, leaving the tip of the toe free.
3 Cut about six pieces of elastic adhesive tape of varying lengths from 6cm to 10cm.
4 Apply the lengths of elastic adhesive tape from the tip of the toe to the base in a figure-of-eight fashion, forming a 'V' from the nail and over the first metatarsal. Snip the tape as required.
5 Apply a length of elastic adhesive tape around the foot to anchor the ends of the tape: leave a 2cm gap to avoid constriction. (Figure **75**)
6 Ensure the circulation is satisfactory: check the colour and warmth of the toe.

## Advice to patients
Keep the spica dry.
If the toe becomes discoloured or numb, or severe pain or tingling develop, return to hospital.
Wear the spica for as long as the doctor advises.
Elevate the foot when sitting or lying down.

**75**

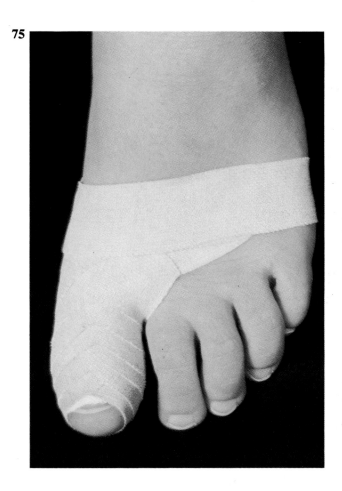

# 29 Dry dressing

## Use
To protect a broken skin surface.

## Equipment
a) Sterile dressing pack, comprising:
   Four pairs of non-toothed forceps
   Gallipot
   Paper towels
   Gauze
   Cotton wool balls
   Tray
b) Non-adherent absorbent dressing.
c) Permeable adhesive tape, 1.25cm width.
d) Elastic adhesive tape, 2.5cm width.
e) Cotton conforming bandage.
f) Scissors.

## Procedure
1 Wound toilet will have been performed already (see page 70). (Figure **76**)
2 Using an aseptic technique, place the non-adherent absorbent dressing, shiny side downwards, on to the wound.
3 Fix the absorbent dressing with permeable adhesive tape, ensuring that the tape does not encircle the whole limb or torso by leaving a gap between the ends to prevent constriction. (Figure **77**)
4 If there is likely to be excessive exudate from the wound, extra gauze may be applied over the absorbent dressing and taped down with permeable adhesive tape.
5 Cover the dressing with conforming bandage around the limb or trunk and secure the bandage with elastic adhesive tape. (Figure **78**)

## Advice to patients
Keep the dressing dry.
If a large amount of blood, pus or fluid appears through the dressing, return to hospital.
Follow the doctor's instructions on how long the dressing is to be worn and whether elevation of the limb is required.

**76**

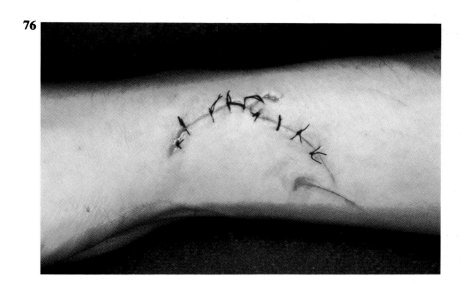

**77**

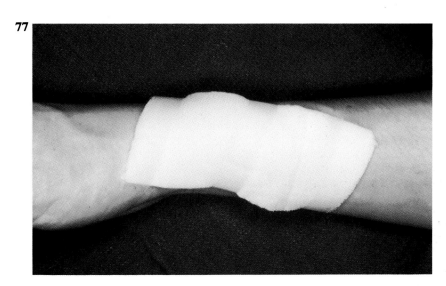

**78**

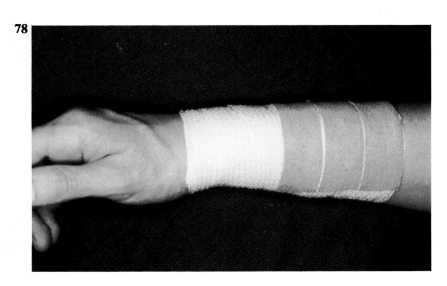

# 30 Pressure dressing: (A) to the head

## Uses
1 To arrest haemorrhage.
2 To prevent formation of haematoma.

## Equipment
a) Sterile dressing pack, comprising:
    Four pairs of non-toothed forceps
    Gallipot
    Paper towels
    Gauze
    Cotton wool balls
    Tray
b) Non-adherent absorbent dressing.
c) Permeable adhesive tape, 1.25cm width.
d) Elastic adhesive tape, 2.5cm width.
e) Crepe bandage.
f) Scissors.

## Procedure
1 The affected area will have been shaved already and wound toilet will have been performed (see page 70). The wound may have been sutured.
2 Using an aseptic technique, place the non-adherent absorbent dressing, shiny side downwards, on to the wound. Place several layers of gauze over the non-adherent dressing. Tape down with permeable adhesive tape, if necessary.
3 Cover the dressing with a crepe bandage applied firmly around the head and secure the crepe bandage with elastic adhesive tape. (Figures **79, 80**)
4 Ensure the patient is accompanied by a relative or friend when discharged.

### Advice to patients
Keep the dressing dry.
If there is excessive bleeding appearing through the dressing, return to hospital.
Leave the dressing in position for at least 24 hours.

---

# 31 Pressure dressing: (B) to a limb

## Uses
1 To arrest haemorrhage.
2 To prevent formation of haematoma.

## Equipment
a) Sterile dressing pack, comprising:
    Four pairs of non-toothed forceps
    Gallipot
    Paper towels
    Gauze
    Cotton wool balls
    Tray
b) Non-adherent absorbent dressing.
c) Permeable adhesive tape, 1.25cm width.
d) Elastic adhesive tape, 2.5cm width.
e) Crepe bandage.
f) Scissors.

## Procedure
1 Wound toilet will have been performed already (see page 70).
2 Using an aseptic technique, place the non-adherent absorbent dressing, shiny side downwards, on to the wound. Place several layers of gauze over the non-adherent dressing. Tape down with permeable adhesive tape, ensuring that the tape does not encircle the whole limb, to prevent constriction. (Figure **81**)
3 Cover the dressing with a crepe bandage applied firmly around the limb and secure the crepe bandage with elastic adhesive tape. (Figure **82**)

### Advice to patients
Keep the dressing dry.
If there is excessive bleeding appearing through the dressing, return to hospital.
Leave the dressing in position for at least 24 hours, elevating the leg or keeping the arm in a sling during this time.

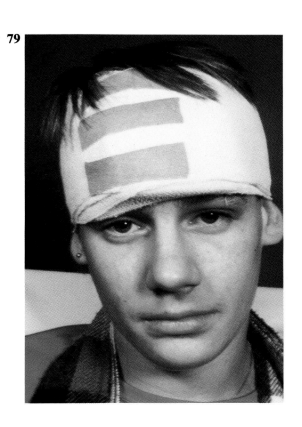

**79**

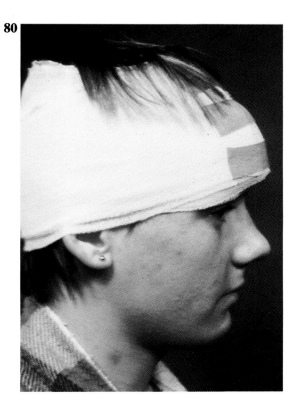

**80**

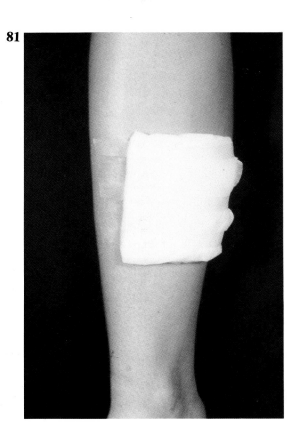

**81**

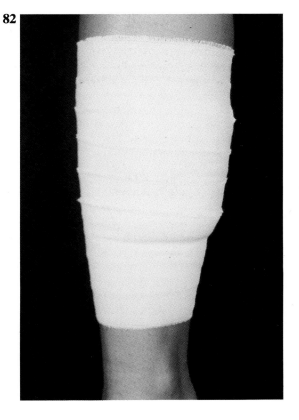

**82**

# 32 Pressure dressing: (C) to a finger

## Use
To arrest haemorrhage from an injured finger.

## Equipment
a) Sterile dressing pack, comprising:
> Four pairs of non-toothed forceps
> Gallipot
> Paper towels
> Gauze
> Cotton wool balls
> Tray

b) Non-adherent absorbent dressing.
c) Permeable adhesive tape, 1.25cm width.
d) Cotton tubular bandage.
e) Applicator for cotton tubular bandage.
f) Elastic adhesive tape, 2.5cm width.
g) Scissors.

## Procedure
1 Wound toilet will have been performed already (see page 70). The wound may have been sutured.
2 Using an aseptic technique, place the non-adherent absorbent dressing, shiny side downwards, on to the wound. Place several layers of gauze over the non-adherent dressing. Tape down with permeable adhesive tape, ensuring that the tape does not completely encircle the finger, to prevent constriction. (Figure **83**)
3 Select the appropriate size of cotton tubular bandage and cut a length about ten times as long as the injured finger. Thread the bandage over the applicator.
4 Pass the applicator over the finger and ease off the end of the bandage; twist the applicator around the base of the finger to anchor the bandage.
5 Twist the applicator continually while retracting it to the end of the finger, in order to give added pressure. At the end of the finger, twist the bandage through two complete turns. (Figure **84**)
6 Repeat steps 4 and 5 until the finger has been covered four times.
7 Split the remaining piece of bandage into two and use the two ends to tie the dressing loosely in position at the base of the finger.
8 Anchor the bandage to the skin at the base of the finger with elastic adhesive tape (Figure **85**). Check that the patient is not allergic to elastic adhesive tape: if so, substitute a non-allergenic tape.
An alternative method of securing the dressing, useful for children, is shown in Figure **86**.
9 Apply a high sling (see page 30).

## Advice to patients
Keep the dressing dry.
If there is excessive bleeding appearing through the dressing, return to hospital.
Leave the dressing in position for at least 24 hours, after which it is replaced by an ordinary finger dressing (see page 66).

**83**

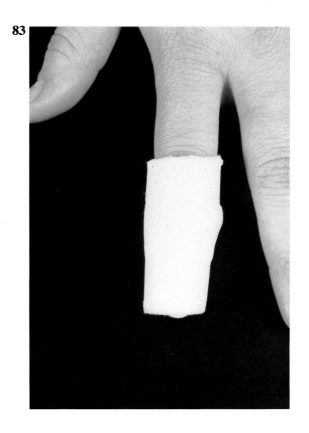

**84**

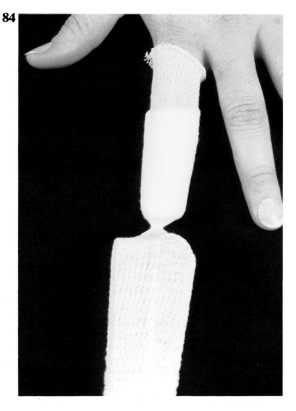

**85**

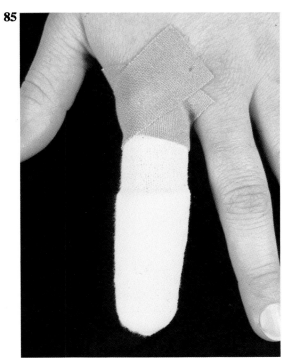

**86**

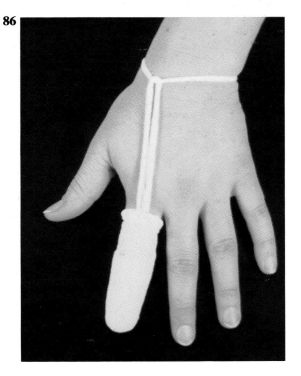

# 33 Burns dressing: (A) to the face, using oxytetracycline and hydrocortisone spray

## Use
To promote healing and prevent infection following a burn or scald of the face.

## Equipment
a) Sterile dressing pack, comprising:
      Four pairs of non-toothed forceps
      Gallipot
      Paper towels
      Gauze
      Cotton wool balls
      Tray
b) Cleansing solution.
c) Sterile needle.
d) Sterile scissors.
e) Oxytetracycline 0.5%, hydrocortisone 0.17% spray.
f) Masks.

## Procedure
N.B. Aseptic technique must be used.
1 Position the patient lying down in comfort.
2 Clean the area of the burn with cleansing solution.
3 Either pop the blisters with a sterile needle and drain the fluid, or remove the top of the blisters with sterile scissors, according to the doctor's instructions.
4 Gently cut away any loose skin, using sterile scissors.
5 Dry the area completely with gauze.
6 Cover the patient's eyes, nose and mouth. Cover his clothes to prevent staining. Tell him to hold his breath.
7 Spray oxytetracycline and hydrocortisone spray over the area of the burn, holding the can about 15cm from the patient's face. (Figures **87, 88**)

## Advice to patients
Keep the area clean and dry.
If the area becomes very painful or inflamed, return to hospital.
Re-apply the spray, according to the doctor's instructions.

**87**

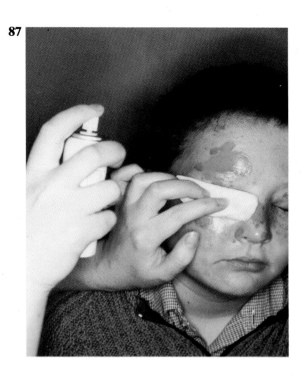

**88**

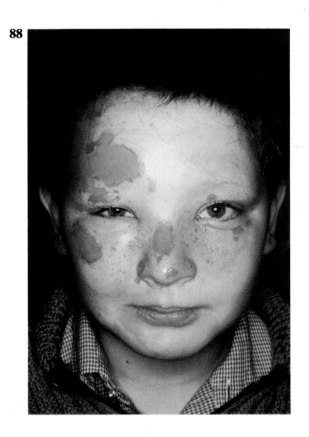

# 34  Burns dressing: (B) to the chest, using povidone-iodine ointment

## Use
To promote healing and prevent infection following a burn or scald of the chest.

## Equipment
a)  Sterile dressing pack, comprising:
      Four pairs of non-toothed forceps
      Gallipot
      Paper towels
      Gauze
      Cotton wool balls
      Tray
b)  Cleansing solution.
c)  Sterile needle.
d)  Sterile scissors.
e)  Povidone-iodine 10% ointment.
f)  Non-adherent absorbent dressing.
g)  Permeable adhesive tape, 1.25cm width.
h)  Cotton conforming bandage.
i)  Elastic adhesive tape, 2.5cm width.
j)  Elastic net bandage.
k)  Masks.

## Procedure
*N.B.* Aseptic technique must be used.
1  Position the patient in comfort, stripped to the waist.
2  A nitrous oxide/oxygen mixture can be used to relieve pain (see page 126).
3  Clean the area of the burn with cleansing solution.
4  Either pop the blisters with a sterile needle and drain the fluid, or remove the top of the blisters with sterile scissors, according to the doctor's instructions.
5  Gently cut away any loose skin, using sterile scissors.
6  Dry the area completely with gauze. (Figure **89**)
7  Spread the povidone-iodine ointment over the affected area, using a piece of gauze. Warn the patient that the ointment may sting at first. (Figure **90**)
8  Cover the area with non-adherent absorbent dressing and gauze and secure with permeable adhesive tape.
9  Bandage the dressing in position, using cotton conforming bandage, secured with elastic adhesive tape. (Figure **91**)
10  Make a vest, using elastic net bandage as follows: cut a piece of elastic net bandage about 40cm long; cut a 1cm hole in each side of the bandage about 10cm from the upper end, for the arms; place the vest over the patient's head, with his arms through the holes; position the vest comfortably and ensure that it secures the whole dressing. (Figure **92**)

## Advice to patients
Keep the dressing dry.
If the area becomes very painful or inflamed, return to hospital.

**89**

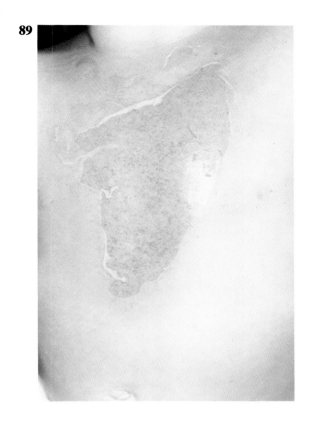

**90**

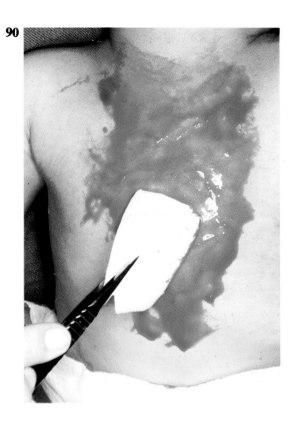

**91**

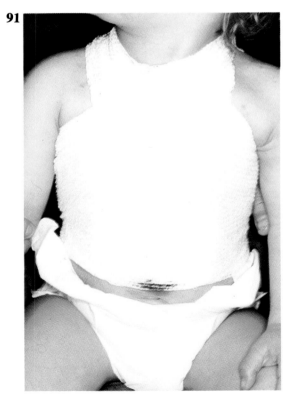

**92**

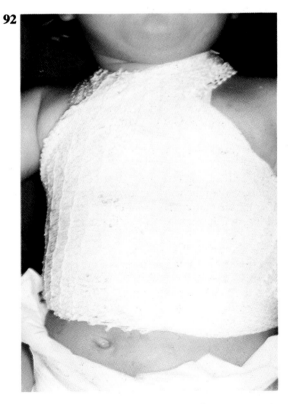

## 35 Burns dressing: (C) to a hand, using silver sulphadiazine and a burn bag

### Use
To promote healing and prevent infection following a burn or scald of the hand.

### Equipment
a) Sterile dressing pack, comprising:
      Four pairs of non-toothed forceps
      Gallipot
      Paper towels
      Gauze
      Cotton wool balls
      Tray
b) Cleansing solution.
c) Sterile needle.
d) Sterile scissors.
e) Silver sulphadiazine 1% cream.
f) Burn bag.
g) Cotton conforming bandage, 7.5cm width.
h) Elastic adhesive tape, 2.5cm width.
i) Mask.

### Procedure
*N.B.* Aseptic technique must be used.
1. Position the patient in comfort with the affected hand and forearm exposed. (Figures **93, 94**)
2. A nitrous oxide/oxygen mixture can be used to relieve pain (see page 126).
3. Clean the area of the burn with cleansing solution.
4. Either pop the blisters with a sterile needle and drain the fluid, or remove the top of the blisters with sterile scissors, according to the doctor's instructions.
5. Gently cut away any loose skin, using sterile scissors.
6. Dry the area completely with gauze.
7. Spread the silver sulphadiazine cream over the area of the burn, using a cotton wool ball, so that the cream is about 4mm thick. (Figure **95**)
8. Apply the burn bag over the entire hand and wrist, ensuring that full mobility of the hand is possible inside the bag.
9. Anchor the burn bag with a cotton conforming bandage around the wrist and secure with elastic adhesive tape. (Figure **96**)
10. Apply a high sling (see page 30).

### Advice to patients
Keep the dressing dry.
If the hand becomes very painful or inflamed, return to hospital.
Fluid will accumulate in the bag; do not burst the bag, as infection could result.
Elevate the limb in the sling, as instructed by the doctor.
Exercise the fingers inside the bag, to prevent stiffness.

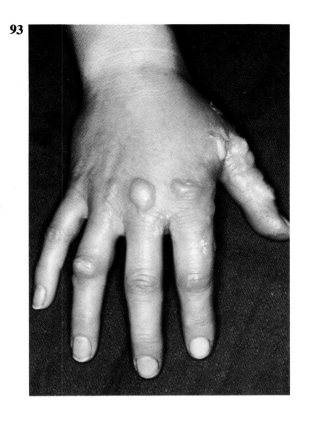

**93**

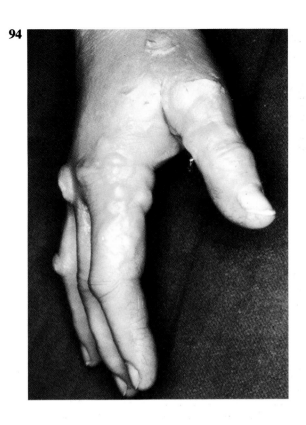

**94**

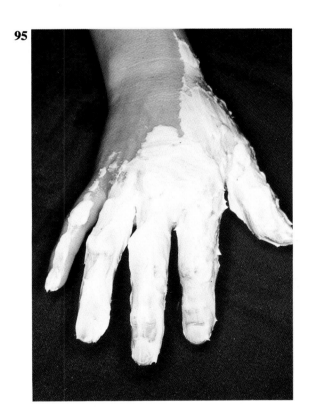

**95**

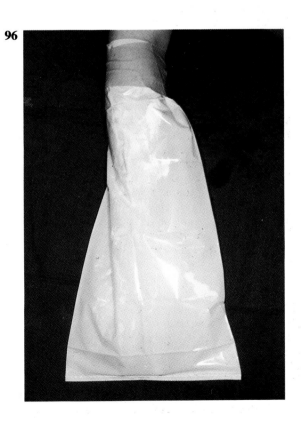

**96**

# 36 Finger/toe dressing

## Uses
1 To protect a broken skin surface on a finger or toe.
2 Following suturing of a finger or toe.

## Equipment
*a)* Sterile dressing pack, comprising:
      Four pairs of non-toothed forceps
      Gallipot
      Paper towels
      Gauze
      Cotton wool balls
      Tray
*b)* Non-adherent absorbent dressing.
*c)* Permeable adhesive tape, 1.25cm width.
*d)* Cotton tubular bandage.
*e)* Applicator for cotton tubular bandage.
*f)* Elastic adhesive tape, 2.5cm width.
*g)* Scissors.

## Procedure
1 Wound toilet will have been performed already (see page 70). The wound may have been sutured.
2 Using aseptic technique, place the non-adherent absorbent dressing, shiny side downwards, on to the wound. Tape down with permeable adhesive tape, ensuring that the tape does not completely encircle the digit, to prevent constriction. (Figure **97**)
3 Cut a length of cotton tubular bandage about five times as long as the injured digit. Thread the bandage over the applicator.
4 Pass the applicator over the digit and ease off the end of the bandage; twist the applicator around the base of the digit, to anchor the bandage.
5 Retract the applicator to the end of the digit and twist the bandage through two complete turns. (Figure **98**)
6 Repeat steps 4 and 5.
7 Split the remaining piece of bandage into two and use the two ends to tie the dressing loosely in position at the base of the digit. (Figure **99**)
8 Anchor the bandage to the skin at the base of the digit with elastic adhesive tape (Figures **100,101**). Check that the patient is not allergic to elastic adhesive tape: if so, substitute a non-allergenic tape.

## Advice to patients
Keep the dressing dry.
If there is excessive bleeding or pus appearing through the dressing, return to hospital.
Follow the doctor's instructions on how long the dressing is to be worn and whether elevation of the limb is necessary.
The digit can be moved as much as the dressing will allow.

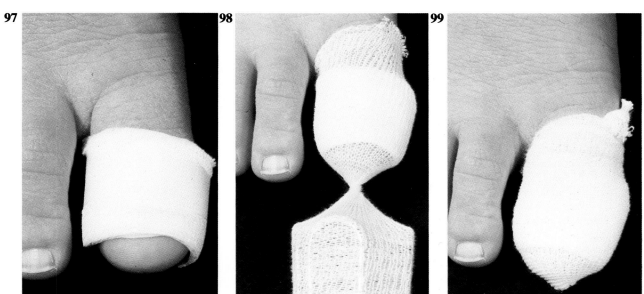

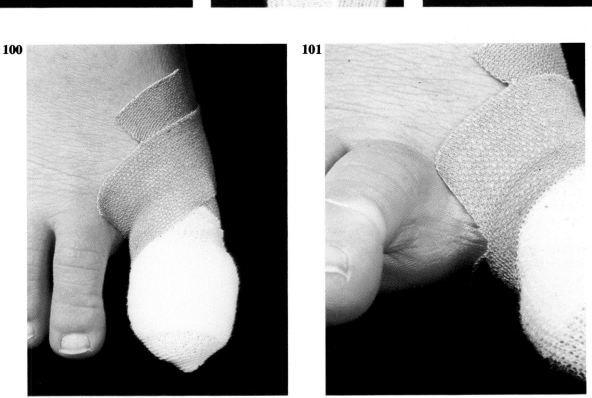

# 37 Skin-closure strips

## Use
To approximate the wound edges in a superficial laceration.

## Equipment
a) Sterile dressing pack, comprising:
> Four pairs of non-toothed forceps
> Gallipot
> Paper towels
> Gauze
> Cotton wool balls
> Tray
b) Cleansing solution.
c) Sterile skin-closure strips.
d) Plastic dressing or tincture of benzoin spray.
e) Scissors.

## Procedure
1 Explain the procedure to the patient.
2 Position the patient in comfort and expose the affected area.
3 Using aseptic technique, swab the wound until it is clean.
4 Thoroughly dry the area with gauze. (Figure **102**).
5 Remove the protective backing from the skin-closure strips.
6 Begin wound-closure at the middle of the wound. Apply a strip to one side of the wound, pressing it firmly into position; approximate the wound edges and continue the application of the strip over the wound and on to the other side of the wound, again pressing firmly into position. (Figure **103**)
7 Position other strips in the same way, leaving about a 3mm gap between strips, until the wound is closed. (Figure **104**)
8 It may be necessary to apply further strips parallel to the wound, to prevent the edges from lifting. Plastic dressing or tincture of benzoin spray applied to the area around the wound makes the skin tacky and the strips adhere more easily.
9 Apply a dry dressing (see page 54) unless the doctor requests otherwise.

## Advice to patients
Keep the wound clean and dry.
If the wound begins to gape or ooze excessively, return to hospital.
The skin-closure strips will be removed by the doctor.

**102**

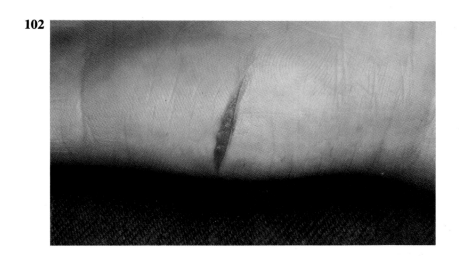

**103**

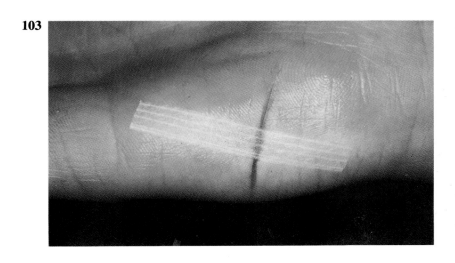

**104**

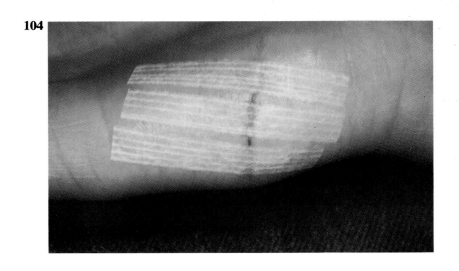

# 38 Wound toilet

## Use
To clean a wound.

*N.B.* In an Accident and Emergency Department, the
nature of the injuries may prevent the use of a strict
aseptic technique. However, all wounds must be
cleaned as thoroughly as possible.
Occasionally, local anaesthesia is needed for
adequate wound toilet.

## Equipment
*a)* Sterile dressing pack, comprising:
Four pairs of non-toothed forceps
Gallipot
Paper towels
Gauze
Cotton wool balls — *there are no longer used due to cotton filaments being left in wounds*
Tray
*b)* Cleansing solution.

## Procedure
1 Explain the procedure to the patient.
2 Position the patient in comfort and expose the
affected area.
3 Using aseptic technique as far as possible, swab the
wound until it is clean. (Figure **105**)
4 Thoroughly dry the area with gauze.
5 Cover the area with a sterile paper towel.
6 The wound may be dressed, sutured or skin-closure
strips applied, according to the nature of the wound
and the doctor's instructions.

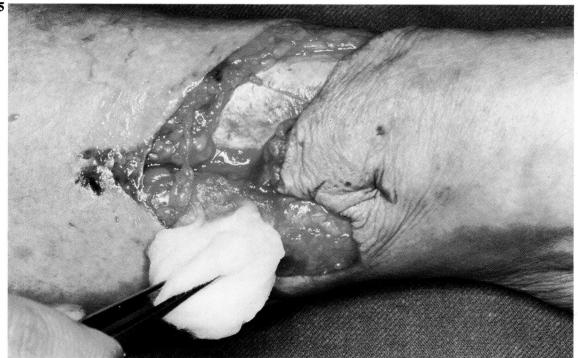

# 39  Packing of wounds

## Use
To allow an infected wound to heal from its base upwards by antiseptic wick insertion.

## Equipment
*a)*  Sterile dressing pack, comprising:
      Four pairs of non-toothed forceps
      Gallipot
      Paper towels
      Gauze
      Cotton wool balls
      Tray
*b)*  Cleansing solution.
*c)*  Ribbon gauze.
*d)*  Topical antiseptic solution (Eusol or proflavine cream).
*e)*  Extra gallipot.
*f)*  Sterile scissors.

## Procedure
1  A nitrous oxide/oxygen mixture can be used to relieve pain (see page 126).
2  Explain the procedure to the patient.
3  Position the patient in comfort and expose the affected area.
4  Using aseptic technique, swab the wound until it is clean.
5  Thoroughly dry the area with gauze. (Figure **106**)
6  Pour some topical antiseptic solution into a gallipot.
7  Using forceps, soak the ribbon gauze in the topical antiseptic solution.
8  Insert one end of the soaked ribbon gauze into the wound, then gently fold it all in, completely packing the wound. (Figures **107,108**)
9  The ribbon gauze can be packed tightly or loosely, according to the doctor's instructions.
10  Cover the wound with gauze and apply a dry dressing (see page 54).

## Advice to patients
Keep the dressing clean and dry.
If there is excessive leakage, return to hospital.

**106**

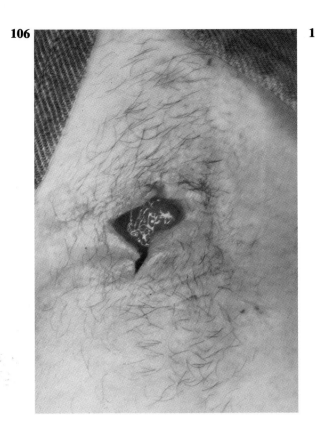

**107**

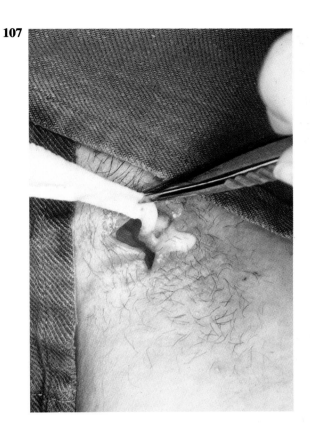

**108**

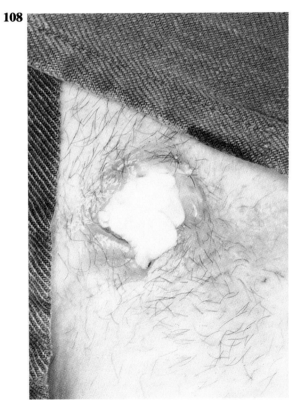

# 40 Topical antiseptic solutions

**Eusol** (Edinburgh University Solution Of Lime)

1 An antiseptic solution containing chlorinated lime 1.25% and boric acid 1.25% in water.

2 Must be freshly prepared and undiluted.

3 Used for packing wounds or for cleaning wounds and ulcers, when it may be applied as a wet dressing. (Figures **109,110**)

4 Effective against both Gram positive and Gram negative bacteria and against spores.

5 Can bleach fabrics.

6 Can be an irritant.

*NO LONGER USED however some consultants will still ask for this*

## Hydrogen peroxide solution

1 A colourless antiseptic solution: most often used as a 6% solution in water and this will release twenty times its own volume of oxygen. This strength is also known as 20-volume strength; solutions stronger than 6% must be diluted before use.

2 Used for cleaning infected wounds and ulcers. It bubbles when it comes into contact with the tissues and oxygen is released. (Figures **111,112**)

3 Helps to separate discharges and is effective against all organisms, both aerobic and anaerobic. It potentiates povidone-iodine by increasing the release of available iodine.

4 Bleaches fabrics.

## Proflavine cream

1 A bright yellow antiseptic cream.

2 Used for packing wounds (Figures **113,114**) and for infected ulcers.

3 Effective against both Gram positive and Gram negative bacteria but not against spores.

4 Not inactivated by body fluids or pus.

5 Non-irritating and non-toxic but stains clothes.

## Silver sulphadiazine cream

1 An antiseptic cream containing 1% silver sulphadiazine.

2 Used for burns (Figures **115,116**, wounds, infected leg ulcers and skin graft donor sites.

3 Effective against both Gram positive and Gram negative bacteria but not against spores. It is particularly effective against *Pseudomonas*.

4 Is applied in a layer about 4mm thick.

5 Occasionally causes hypersensitivity and leucopenia.

6 Contraindicated in pregnancy or in infants under three months old, and in patients who are sensitive to sulphonamides.

7 Should be used with caution if there is impaired kidney or liver function.

*\* Not suitable as a primary dressing if being referred to a burns unit. Use paraffin gauze in multiple layers so that they can assess burn damage.*

## Povidone-iodine ointment

1 An antiseptic ointment containing 10% povidone-iodine.

2 Used for burns (Figures **117,118**) and wounds.

3 Effective against all bacterial species and against spores, fungi and viruses.

4 Sensitivity is rare.

5 Can stain clothes.

*Take care with thyroid deficient patients.*

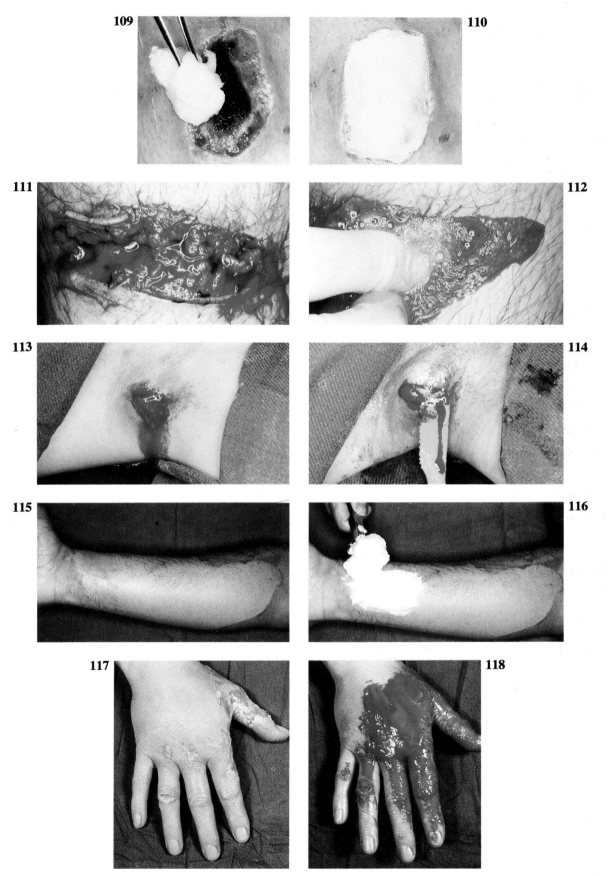

# 41 Plasters

Plaster of Paris is hemihydrated calcium sulphate. When mixed with water, it forms hydrated calcium sulphate and heat is given off. Plaster of Paris bandages are available as rolls or as slabs. The techniques described here use rolls. Other types of external splintage are available: some dry more rapidly (Figure **119**); some are lighter in weight; some are more radiolucent; some do not disintegrate in water. Plaster of Paris is most frequently used.

## PREPARATION OF THE PATIENT

1 Before applying the Plaster of Paris, establish exactly how the doctor wants the limb to be positioned. The patient may be required to sit on a chair or lie on a trolley or plaster table, depending upon the area injured.
2 Explain the treatment to the patient before applying the plaster.
3 Plasters are often applied while the patient is anaesthetised, after the fracture has been manipulated.
4 For above-elbow plasters, above-knee plasters and plaster cylinders, expose the entire limb.
5 All jewellery must be removed from the injured limb and not replaced while the plaster is in use.
6 When applying plaster, protect the patient's clothing with a plastic sheet.
7 Any lacerations or abrasions must be cleaned and dressed before the cotton tubular bandage/ orthopaedic wool is applied; their positions must be noted in case there is wound leakage.
8 Particular care must be taken when a plaster is applied over the elbow or knee, to avoid constriction.

## APPLICATION OF ORTHOPAEDIC WOOL

This must be wrapped around the limb smoothly, evenly and without wrinkles. It is designed to be eased and stretched around the body contours and over bony prominences. Very swollen areas and bony prominences should be protected by a double layer of wool.

## APPLICATION OF PLASTER OF PARIS BANDAGES

1 The water to be used should be luke-warm, never hot. The warmer the water, the quicker the plaster sets.
2 Holding the end of the bandage in one hand and the roll of bandage in the other hand, immerse the bandage in the water until it stops bubbling.
3 Lift out the bandage and squeeze it gently to remove excess water.
4 Apply the bandage around the limb, covering two-thirds of the width of the previous turn each time. Smooth it over body contours and bony prominences. It may be necessary to pleat the bandage to do this.
5 Each bandage must be moulded firmly and carefully to prevent air from collecting between the layers, which would weaken the final plaster.

6 The plaster must be of equal thickness over its whole length; unequal thicknesses would weaken the final plaster.
7 A full plaster completely encircles the limb. A plaster slab covers only part of the circumference of the limb. Swelling of the limb, therefore, is more likely to endanger the circulation with a full plaster than with a plaster slab. A plaster slab can be removed more rapidly in an emergency.
8 A full plaster may be split (i.e. cut along its length) immediately after application, using a plaster knife (or shears). Cut down through the plaster to the wool along the full length of the plaster. Swelling is much less likely to endanger the circulation if the plaster is split; also, wounds can be inspected.
9 A full plaster can be bivalved (i.e. split along both sides); if the top section is removed, a backslab remains and can be secured in position with a crepe bandage. A backslab also can be made directly.
10 Remove any excess plaster from the patient's skin after applying the plaster.

## REMOVAL OF PLASTER OF PARIS

1 Reassure the patient when using an electric plaster saw; it is noisy and looks dangerous.
2 The blade of an electric plaster saw oscillates forwards and back; it does not rotate. It can cut the skin and must be used with care. There must be a layer of orthopaedic wool between the plaster and the skin.
3 Press the blade of the saw downwards on to the plaster: when the plaster has been sawn through, the nurse feels a 'give'. Repeat this action along the entire length of the plaster but avoid the extreme ends, which should be cut with plaster shears. Avoid leaving the saw in one place for more than a few seconds as it generates heat. The cutting movement is up and down, not sideways. (Figures **120,121**)
4 Keep hands dry when using an electric saw, to avoid an electric shock.
5 Do not use the electric saw near oxygen, to avoid an explosion.
6 When using plaster shears, keep the lower handle parallel to the plaster and move the upper handle up and down. (Figures **122,123**)
7 Push the points of the shears onwards very carefully and, before closing the blades, ensure they are not going to dig into the limb. Particular care is needed near joints.
8 Avoid cutting over a bony prominence or a concavity, if possible.
9 A lower limb plaster can be cut up both sides for easy removal.
10 An upper limb plaster usually can be prised open after being cut along its length.
11 When a plaster has been cut or sawn, the underlying orthopaedic wool can be cut with scissors and the plaster removed. (Figures **124,125**)

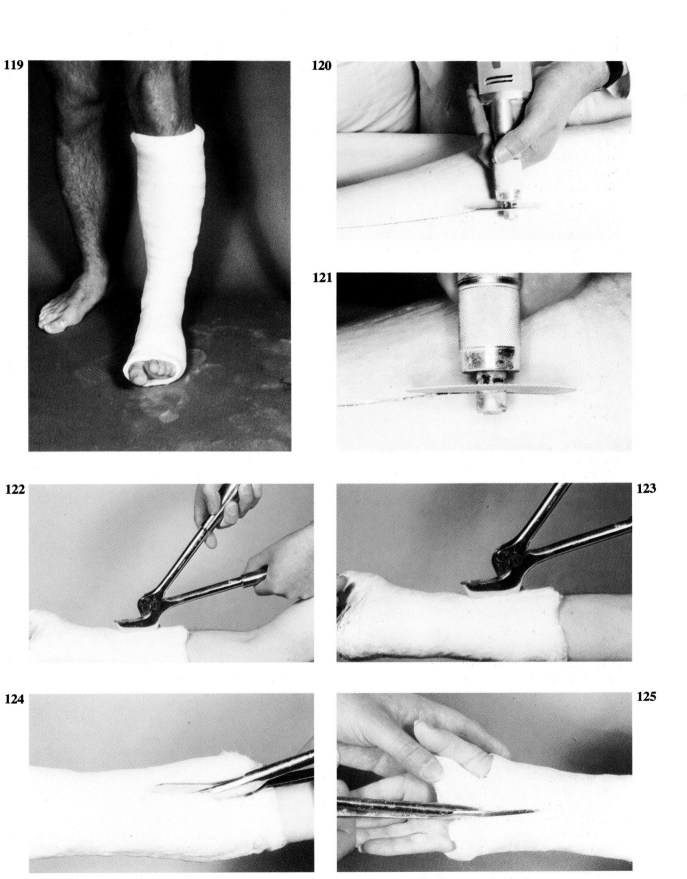

# 42 Instructions for the patient in plaster

1 Return to hospital immediately if the fingers/toes become blue, swollen, very painful, very cold, stiff, red or begin to tingle.
2 Plaster of Paris takes about 48 hours to dry: do not bear weight on the plaster during this time.
3 Elevate the arm or leg on a soft surface (for example, a pillow or sling) while the plaster is drying.
4 If the leg is in plaster, the foot should be higher than the waist when sitting or lying.
5 Do not use a hairdryer or direct heat to dry the plaster, as this causes crumbling.
6 Keep the plaster dry.
7 Do not write on the plaster with a felt-tip pen.
8 Never put anything down the plaster.
9 If the plaster cracks or becomes loose, return to hospital.
10 Exercise the parts of the limb which are not included in the plaster, according to the doctor's instructions. The exercises should be performed for five minutes every hour, during the day.

## EXERCISES
### Upper limb

1 Fully straighten out the fingers and thumb (Figure **126**); then make a tight fist and bend the thumb. (Figure **127**)
2 Spread the fingers wide apart (Figure **128**); then close them together. (Figure **129**)
3 Touch the tip of the thumb to the tip of the little finger (Figure **130**); slide it down the little finger. (Figure **131**)
4 Exercise the shoulder and elbow by removing the arm from the sling, raising both arms above the head (Figure **132**) and circle them to meet behind the back at waist level. (Figure **133**)
5 When the plaster is dry, the arm should be used as normally as possible, according to the doctor's instructions.

### Lower limb

1 Wriggle the toes.
2 Hold the foot at right angles and tighten the muscle at the front of the thigh.
3 Raise the straightened leg for five seconds, then lower it slowly.
4 Rotate the ankle clockwise and anti-clockwise.

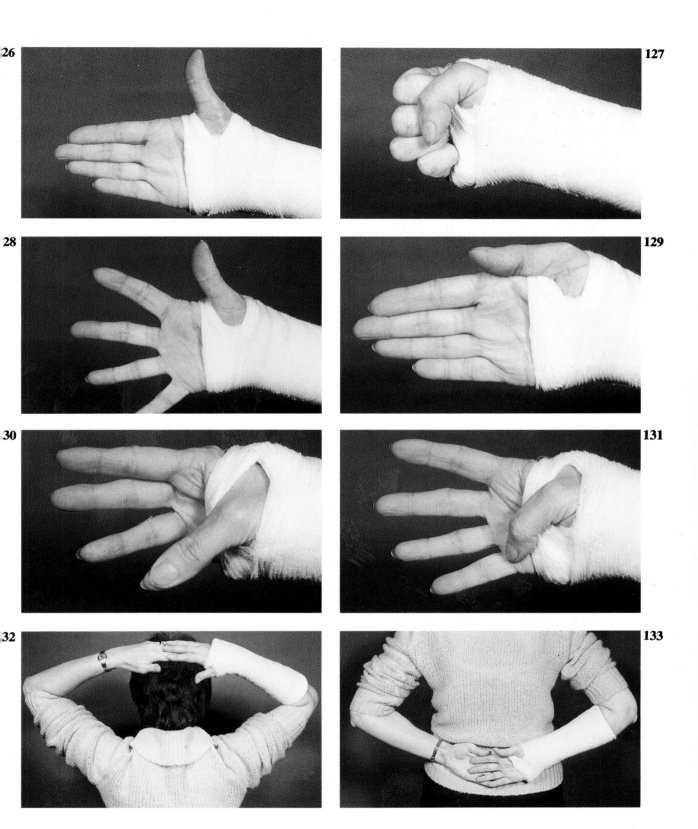

# 43  Above-elbow backslab plaster

## Uses
1  Supracondylar fracture of the humerus.
2  Following reduction of a dislocated elbow.
3  Fracture of the head of the radius.
4  Fracture of the radius and ulna.

## Equipment
*a)*  Orthopaedic wool, 7.5cm width.
*b)*  Orthopaedic wool, 10cm width.
*c)*  Plaster of Paris bandage, 15cm width.
*d)*  Cotton conforming bandage, 10cm width.
*e)*  Scissors.
*f)*  Plastic sheet.
*g)*  Bucket of warm water.

## Procedure
1  Position the patient in comfort on a chair with the injured arm exposed to the shoulder.
2  Protect the patient's clothes with the plastic sheet.
3  Position the arm with the elbow at right angles and the hand in a neutral position.
4  Make a Plaster of Paris slab by folding the plaster bandage seven times, so that the final slab extends from the knuckles to the axilla and consists of eight layers of plaster bandage.
5  Cut a semicircle from one corner of the plaster slab to accommodate the thumb.
6  Apply 7.5cm orthopaedic wool from the knuckles to the elbow and 10cm orthopaedic wool from the elbow to the axilla. (Figure **134**)
7  Immerse the plaster slab in warm water, ensuring that the layers do not separate by holding the ends together.
8  Apply the plaster slab along the posterior surface of the forearm, elbow and upper arm, from the knuckles to just below the axilla.
9  Smooth out all wrinkles.
10  Turn back the excess wool over the plaster slab, ensuring that the knuckles are exposed and the axilla is free.
11  Apply wet cotton conforming bandage in a spiral fashion to anchor the plaster slab in position, ensuring that the bandage does not constrict the elbow crease.
12  Cut a double layer of plaster bandage, 7.5cm × 5cm; immerse it in warm water and use it to anchor the cotton conforming bandage (Figure **135**). Apply it over the plaster slab, not over the wool (which would form a complete plaster and endanger the circulation). (Figure **136**)
13  Apply a broad arm sling (see page 28).

## Advice to patients
Follow instructions and exercises for the upper limb (see page 78).

**134**

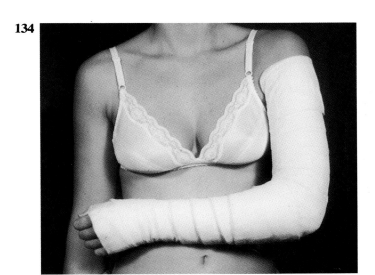

**135**

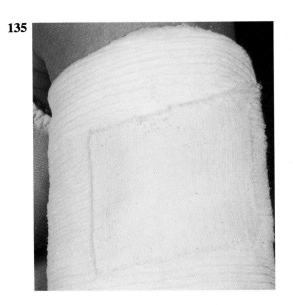

**136**

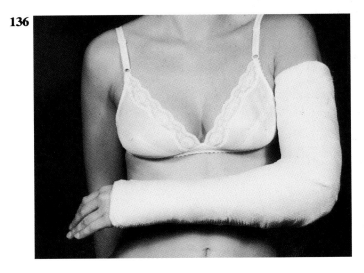

# 44 Below-elbow backslab plaster

## Uses
1 Fracture of the distal radius and ulna.
2 Certain injuries of the bones or soft tissues in the area of the wrist or hand.
3 Inflammation in the area of the wrist or hand (e.g. tenosynovitis).
4 Following surgery in the area of the wrist or hand (e.g. tendon repair).

## Equipment
a) Orthopaedic wool, 7.5cm width.
b) Plaster of Paris bandage, 15cm width.
c) Cotton conforming bandage, 10cm width.
d) Scissors.
e) Plastic sheet.
f) Bucket of warm water.

## Procedure
1 Position the patient in comfort on a chair with the injured arm exposed to above the elbow.
2 Protect the patient's clothes with the plastic sheet.
3 Position the arm with the wrist and hand in a neutral position.
4 Make a Plaster of Paris slab by folding the plaster bandage seven times, so that the final slab extends from the knuckles to 5cm below the elbow and consists of eight layers of plaster bandage.
5 Cut a semicircle from one corner of the plaster slab to accommodate the thumb.
6 Apply the orthopaedic wool from the knuckles to the elbow, leaving the thumb free. (Figure **137**)
7 Immerse the plaster slab in warm water, ensuring that the layers do not separate by holding the ends together.
8 Apply the plaster slab along the posterior surface of the forearm, from the knuckles to just below the elbow. (Figure **138**)
9 Smooth out all wrinkles.
10 Turn back the excess wool over the plaster slab, ensuring that the knuckles are exposed and full elbow movement is possible.
11 Apply wet cotton conforming bandage in a spiral fashion to anchor the plaster slab in position.
12 Cut a double layer of plaster bandage, 7.5cm × 5cm; immerse it in warm water and use it to anchor the cotton conforming bandage. Apply it over the plaster slab, not over the wool (which would form a complete plaster and endanger the circulation). (Figures **139,140**)
13 Apply a broad arm sling (see page 28).

## Advice to patients
Follow instructions and exercises for the upper limb (see page 78).

**137**

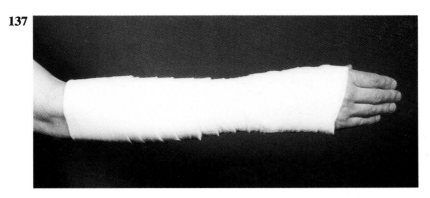

**138**

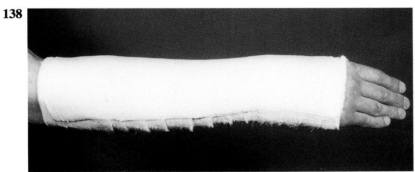

**139**

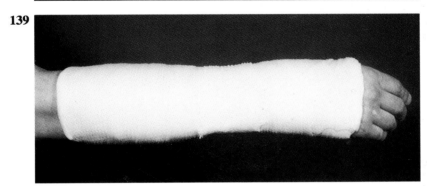

**140**

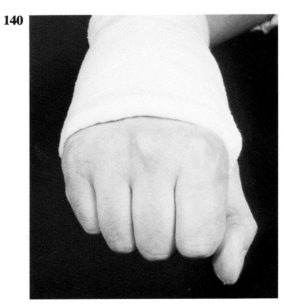

# 45  Plaster for Colles' fracture

## Use
Colles' fracture (a fracture of the lower end of the radius in which the distal fragment is rotated backwards, shifted backwards and tilted to the radial side, producing a 'dinner-fork' deformity).

## Equipment
*a)* Orthopaedic wool, 7.5cm width.
*b)* Plaster of Paris bandage, 7.5cm width.
*c)* Scissors.
*d)* Plastic sheet.
*e)* Bucket of warm water.

## Procedure
1  Position the patient in comfort on a chair with the injured arm exposed to above the elbow.
2  Protect the patient's clothes with the plastic sheet.
3  Position the arm according to the doctor's instructions: usually the wrist is flexed and in ulnar deviation.
4  Apply orthopaedic wool from knuckles to elbow. (Figure **141**)
5  Immerse one roll of Plaster of Paris bandage in warm water.
6  Anchor the plaster bandage around the wrist with two fixing turns; continue around the hand in a figure-of-eight fashion; continue up the forearm in a spiral fashion, covering two-thirds of the width of the bandage with each turn, to the elbow. (This usually requires two plaster bandages.)
7  Smooth out all wrinkles.
8  Turn back the excess wool over the plaster, ensuring that the knuckles are exposed and full elbow movement is possible. (Figure **142**)
9  Neaten the plaster with a third plaster bandage, securing the loose wool. (Figures **143,144**)
10  Apply a broad arm sling (see page 28).

## Advice to patients
Follow instructions and exercises for the upper limb (see page 78).

**141**

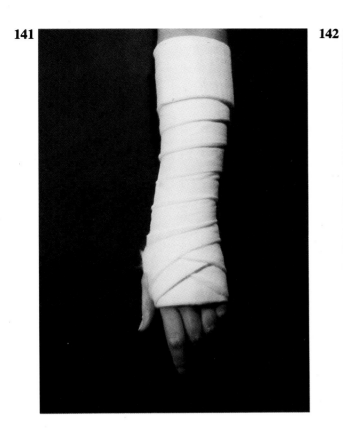

**142**

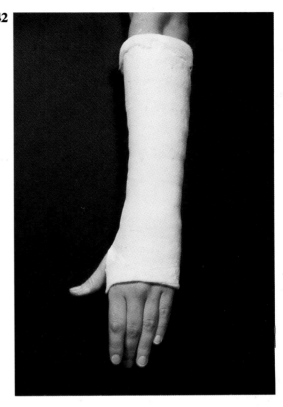

**143**

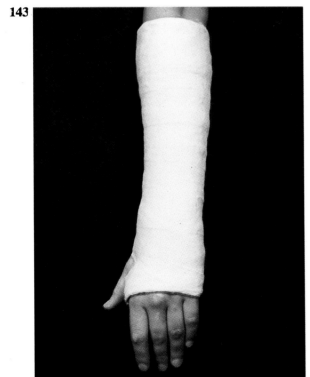

**144**

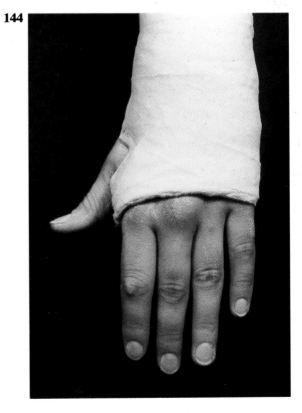

# 46 Plaster for Smith's fracture

## Use
Smith's fracture (a fracture of the lower end of the radius in which the distal fragment is rotated forwards, shifted forwards and tilted to the radial side).

## Equipment
a) Cotton tubular bandage, 7.5cm width.
b) Orthopaedic wool, 7.5cm width.
c) Orthopaedic wool, 10cm width.
d) Plaster of Paris bandage, 7.5cm width.
e) Plaster of Paris bandage, 10cm width.
f) Scissors.
g) Plastic sheet.
h) Bucket of warm water.

## Procedure
1 Position the patient in comfort with the injured arm exposed to the shoulder.
2 Protect the patient's clothes with the plastic sheet.
3 Apply the cotton tubular bandage from the knuckles to the axilla, making a small cut in the bandage to accommodate the thumb. (Figure **145**)
4 The arm is positioned according to the doctor's instructions: usually the forearm is fully supinated and the wrist is extended; the elbow is at right angles.
5 Apply 7.5cm orthopaedic wool from knuckles to elbow and 10cm orthopaedic wool from elbow to axilla. (Figure **146**)
6 Immerse one roll of 7.5cm Plaster of Paris bandage in warm water.
7 Anchor the plaster bandage around the wrist with two fixing turns; continue around the hand in a figure-of-eight fashion; continue up the forearm in a spiral fashion, covering two-thirds of the width of the bandage with each turn, to the elbow. Ensure that the thumb is free.
8 Repeat steps 6 and 7 with a second roll of 7.5cm plaster bandage. (Figure **147**)
9 Immerse one roll of 10cm Plaster of Paris bandage in warm water.
10 Apply the plaster bandage from below the elbow to the axilla, covering two-thirds of the width of the bandage with each turn.
11 Repeat steps 9 and 10 with a second roll of 10cm plaster bandage.
12 Smooth out all wrinkles.
13 Turn back the excess cotton tubular bandage and wool over the plaster, ensuring that the knuckles are exposed and the axilla and the thumb are free. (Figures **148,149**)
14 Neaten the plaster with two more plaster bandages, securing the loose wool and cotton tubular bandage. (Figure **150**)
15 Apply a broad arm sling (see page 28).

## Advice to patients
Follow instructions and exercises for the upper limb (see page 78).

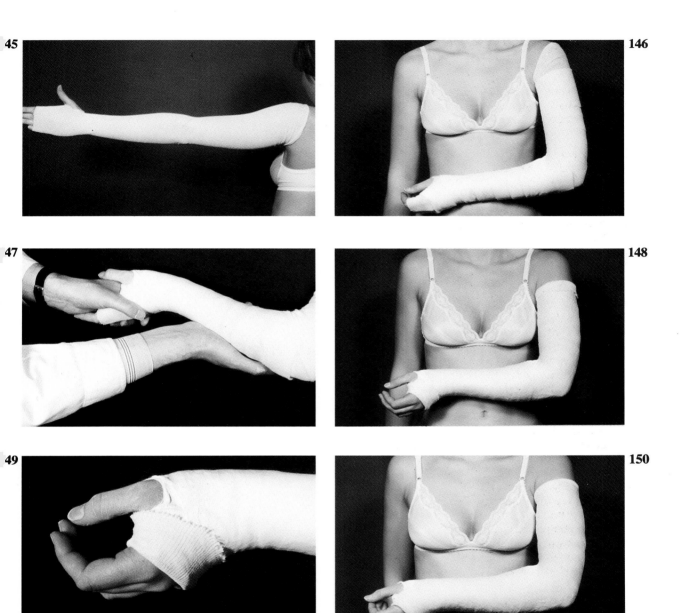

# 47  Plaster for scaphoid fracture

## Uses
1  Fracture of the scaphoid.
2  Suspected fracture of the scaphoid.

## Equipment
*a)*  Cotton tubular bandage, 1.5cm width.
*b)*  Cotton tubular bandage, 5cm width.
*c)*  Orthopaedic wool, 7.5cm width.
*d)*  Plaster of Paris bandage, 7.5cm width.
*e)*  Scissors.
*f)*  Plastic sheet.
*g)*  Bucket of warm water.

## Procedure
1  Seat the patient in comfort on a chair with the injured arm exposed to above the elbow and the elbow resting on the table.
2  Protect the patient's clothes with the plastic sheet.
3  Apply 5cm cotton tubular bandage from knuckles to elbow, making a small hole in the bandage to accommodate the thumb.
4  Apply 1.5cm cotton tubular bandage to the thumb.
5  The arm is positioned according to the doctor's instructions: ask the patient to cock the wrist back and hold an imaginary roll of bandage in the palm of the hand, with the tip of the index finger touching the tip of the thumb. This position must be maintained until the plaster is completed. (Figures **151,152**)
6  Apply orthopaedic wool from knuckles to elbow and around the thumb. (Figure **153**)
7  Immerse one roll of Plaster of Paris bandage in warm water and apply this around the thumb to the interphalangeal joint and around the hand to secure the position of the hand and thumb.
8  Immerse another roll of plaster bandage in warm water and apply this from the wrist to just below the elbow in a spiral fashion, covering two-thirds of the width of the bandage with each turn.
9  Smooth out all wrinkles.
10  Turn back the excess cotton tubular bandage and wool over the plaster, ensuring that the knuckles and the distal half of the thumb and the elbow are free.
11  Neaten the plaster with another roll of plaster bandage, securing the loose wool and cotton tubular bandage. (Figures **154,155**)
12  Apply a broad arm sling (see page 28).

## Advice to patients
Follow instructions and exercises for the upper limb (see page 78).

**151**

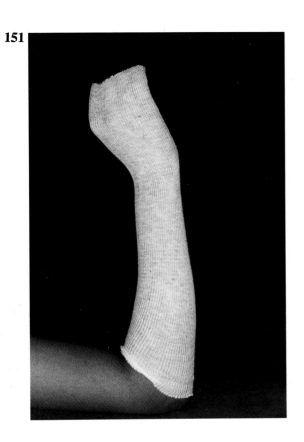

**152**

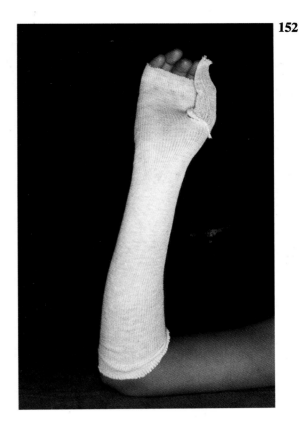

**154**

**153**

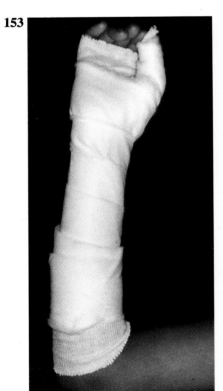

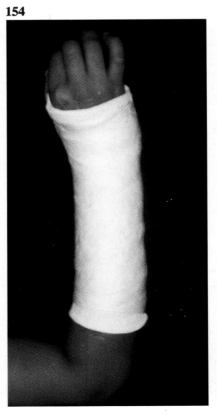

**155**

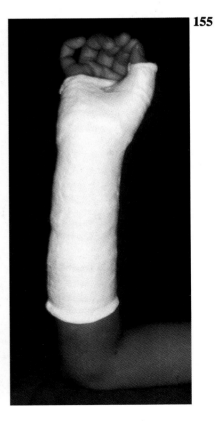

# 48 Above-knee plaster

## Use
Fracture of the tibia and fibula.

## Equipment
a) Cotton tubular bandage, 10cm width.
b) Orthopaedic wool, 10cm width.
c) Orthopaedic wool, 15cm width.
d) Plaster of Paris bandage, 15cm width.
e) Plaster of Paris bandage, 20cm width.
f) Scissors.
g) Plastic sheet.
h) Bucket of warm water.
i) Plaster bridge.

## Procedure
*N.B.* Three nurses are required.

1 Position the patient in comfort on the plaster table with the injured leg exposed to the groin and with the knee supported by the plaster bridge when necessary.
2 Protect the patient's clothes with the plastic sheet.
3 A nurse holds the foot at right angles and maintains this position throughout the procedure.
4 Apply cotton tubular bandage from toes to groin. (Figure **156**)
5 Apply 10cm orthopaedic wool from toes to knee and 15cm orthopaedic wool from knee to groin. (Figure **157**)
6 Immerse one roll of 15cm Plaster of Paris bandage in warm water and apply this from the base of the toes to the ankle. Repeat this procedure with a second roll of 15cm plaster bandage.
7 Immerse a third roll of 15cm Plaster of Paris bandage in warm water and apply this from ankle to knee, in a spiral fashion, pleating it where necessary to accommodate the contours of the limb. Repeat this procedure with a fourth roll of 15cm plaster bandage. (Figure **158**)
8 The plaster bridge is now removed and a nurse maintains the knee in about 10° of flexion throughout the remainder of the procedure.
9 Immerse a fifth roll of 15cm Plaster of Paris bandage in warm water and apply this from below the knee to the mid-thigh, in a spiral fashion. Repeat this procedure with a sixth roll of 15cm plaster bandage.
10 Immerse one roll of 20cm Plaster of Paris bandage in warm water and apply this from above the knee to the groin, in a spiral fashion. Repeat this procedure with a second roll of 20cm plaster bandage.
11 Smooth out all wrinkles.
12 Turn back the excess cotton tubular bandage and wool over the plaster, ensuring that the toes and groin are free. (Figure **159**)
13 Neaten the plaster with two more plaster bandages, applied from toes to groin in a spiral fashion, securing the loose wool and cotton tubular bandage. (Figure **160**)

## Advice to patients
Use the walking aid provided (see page 24).
Follow instructions and exercises for the lower limb (see page 78).

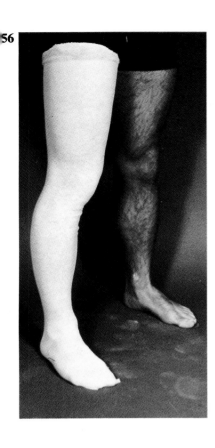

**156**

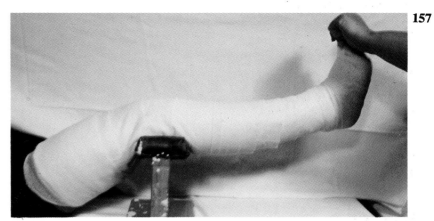

**157**

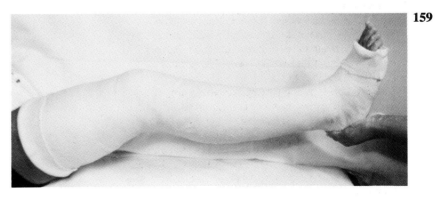

**158**

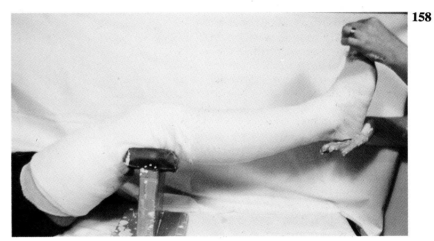

**159**

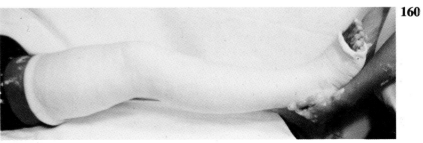

**160**

# 49 Below-knee plaster

## Uses
1 Fracture of the fibula.
2 Certain fractures around the ankle.
3 Certain sprains of the ankle.
4 Certain fractures of the bones of the foot.

## Equipment
*a)* Cotton tubular bandage, 7.5cm width.
*b)* Orthopaedic wool, 10cm width.
*c)* Plaster of Paris bandage, 15cm width.
*d)* Scissors.
*e)* Plastic sheet.
*f)* Bucket of warm water.
*g)* Plaster bridge.

## Procedure
*N.B.* Two nurses are required.
1 Position the patient in comfort on the plaster table with the injured leg exposed to above the knee and with the knee supported by the plaster bridge when necessary.
2 Protect the patient's clothes with the plastic sheet.
3 A nurse holds the foot at right angles and maintains this position throughout the procedure.
4 Apply cotton tubular bandage from toes to knee. (Figure **161**)
5 Apply orthopaedic wool from toes to knee. (Figure **162**)
6 Immerse one roll of Plaster of Paris bandage in warm water and apply this from the base of the toes to the ankle. Repeat this procedure with a second roll of plaster bandage. (Figure **163**)
7 Immerse a third roll of Plaster of Paris bandage in warm water and apply this from ankle to knee, in a spiral fashion. Repeat this procedure with a fourth roll of plaster bandage.
*8 Make a Plaster of Paris slab by folding the plaster bandage seven times, so that the final slab is the length of the foot and consists of eight layers of plaster bandage.
*9 Immerse the plaster slab in warm water, ensuring that the layers do not separate by holding the ends together.
*10 Apply the plaster slab from the base of the toes to the heel and smooth it into position.
11 Smooth out all wrinkles.
12 Turn back the excess cotton tubular bandage and wool over the plaster, ensuring that the toes are free and full knee movement is possible. (Figure **164**)
13 Neaten the plaster with a final roll of plaster bandage, applied from the toes to 5cm below the knee in a spiral fashion; this secures the loose wool and cotton tubular bandage and the foot-piece slab. (Figure **165**)

*Steps 8, 9, 10 are omitted if a non-weight-bearing plaster is required.

## Advice to patients
Use the walking aid provided (see page 24).
Follow instructions and exercises for the lower limb (see page 78).

**161**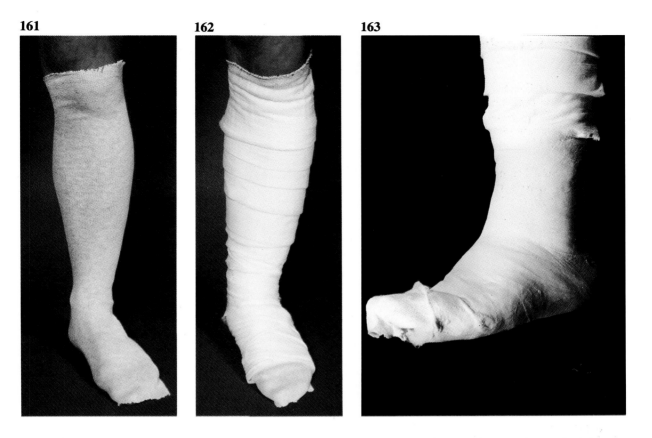

**162**

**163**

**164**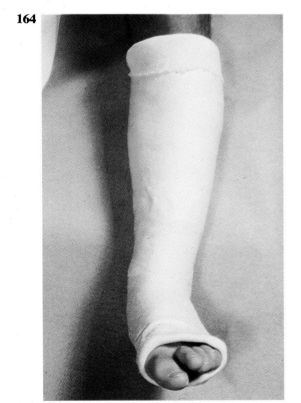

**165**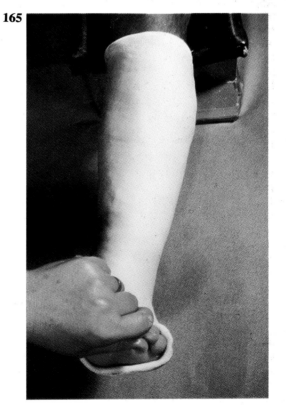

93

# 50  Plaster cylinder

## Uses
1  Fracture of the patella.
2  Following reduction of a dislocated patella.
3  Certain soft tissue injuries of the knee.

## Equipment
*a)*  Cotton tubular bandage, 10cm width.
*b)*  Orthopaedic wool, 10cm width.
*c)*  Orthopaedic wool, 15cm width.
*d)*  Plaster of Paris bandage, 15cm width.
*e)*  Plaster of Paris bandage, 20cm width.
*f)*  Orthopaedic adhesive felt, 1cm thickness.
*g)*  Scissors.
*h)*  Plastic sheet.
*i)*  Bucket of warm water.
*j)*  Plaster bridge.

## Procedure
*N.B.* Two nurses are required.

1  Position the patient in comfort on the plaster table with the injured leg exposed to the groin and with the knee supported by the plaster bridge when necessary.
2  Protect the patient's clothes with the plastic sheet.
3  A nurse lifts the leg by holding the foot.
4  Apply the cotton tubular bandage from ankle to groin (Figure **166**), with the knee straight or slightly flexed, according to the doctor's instructions.
5  Cut a piece of orthopaedic felt about 6cm wide and long enough to encircle the ankle; apply this above the malleoli, encircling the ankle, to prevent the cylinder from slipping down. (Figure **167**)
6  Apply 10cm orthopaedic wool from above the malleoli to the knee and 15cm orthopaedic wool from knee to groin. (Figure **168**)
7  Immerse one roll of 15cm Plaster of Paris bandage in warm water and apply this from above the malleoli to the knee, in a spiral fashion. Repeat this procedure with a second roll of 15cm plaster bandage.
8  The plaster bridge is now removed and a nurse maintains the knee in the required position throughout the remainder of the procedure.
9  Immerse a third roll of 15cm Plaster of Paris bandage in warm water and apply this from below the knee to mid-thigh, in a spiral fashion. Repeat this procedure with a fourth roll of 15cm plaster bandage.
10  Immerse a fifth roll of 15cm Plaster of Paris bandage in warm water and apply this from mid-thigh to groin, in a spiral fashion. Repeat this procedure with a sixth roll of 15cm plaster bandage.
11  Mould the plaster around the knee to prevent it from slipping down.
12  Smooth out all wrinkles.
13  Turn back the excess cotton tubular bandage and wool over the plaster, ensuring that full ankle and hip movements are possible. (Figure **169**)
14  Neaten the plaster with a roll of 20cm Plaster of Paris bandage, applied over the length of the cylinder in a spiral fashion, securing the loose wool and cotton tubular bandage. (Figures **170,171**)

## Advice to patients
Use the walking aid provided (see page 24).
Follow instructions and exercises for the lower limb (see page 78).

**166**

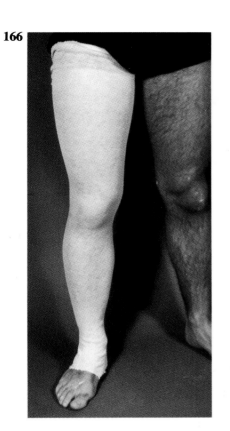

**167**

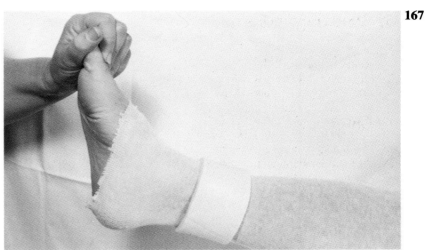

**168**

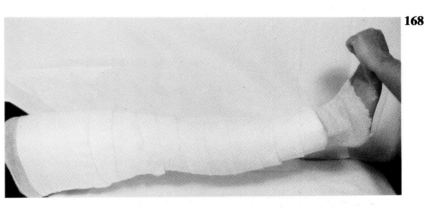

**170**

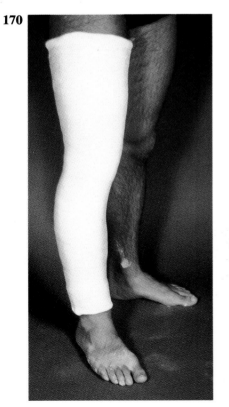

**169**

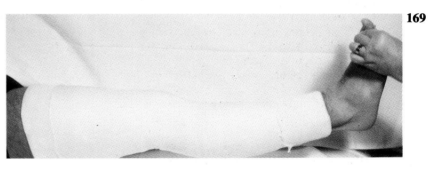

**171**

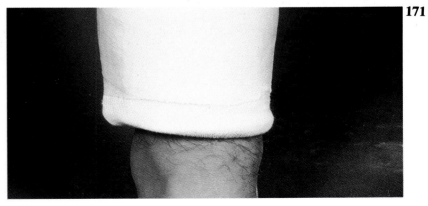

95

# 51  Venous blood sampling

## Use
To obtain a specimen of venous blood for laboratory analysis.

## Equipment
a) Syringe, large enough for the volume of blood required.
b) Sterile needle, 21 gauge.
c) Alcohol-impregnated swab.
d) Tourniquet.
e) Bottle(s) for the blood.
f) Laboratory request card(s).
g) Name labels.
h) Receiver.
i) Elastic adhesive wound dressing.

## Procedure
1 Ensure the correct bottle(s) and request card(s) are available.
2 Explain the procedure to the patient. Position him sitting or lying down in comfort and expose his arm, from above the elbow to the hand.
3 Apply the tourniquet above the elbow and ask the patient to open and close his fist a few times, to engorge the veins with blood.
4 The doctor swabs the area and withdraws the blood (Figure **172**). He then removes the tourniquet and places the swab over the puncture site before removing the needle from the arm. He puts the blood into the bottle(s).
5 Apply pressure over the puncture site until bleeding stops, then apply an adhesive wound dressing.
6 Ensure the bottle(s) are labelled, put them in a receiver and send them to the laboratory with the request card(s).

---

# 52  Arterial blood sampling

## Use
To obtain a specimen of arterial blood for laboratory analysis of blood gases and acid/base balance.

## Equipment
a) Syringe.
b) Two sterile needles, 21 gauge.
c) Alcohol-impregnated swabs.
d) Heparin (5000i.u./ml).
e) Cap for syringe.
f) Laboratory request card.
g) Name labels.
h) Receiver.
i) Ice.
j) Elastic adhesive wound dressing.

## Procedure
1 Ensure that the laboratory is ready to receive the specimen immediately.
2 Explain the procedure to the patient. Position him lying down in comfort. Check whether the doctor will use the radial artery at the wrist or the femoral artery in the groin and expose the appropriate area.
3 Draw up 1ml of heparin into the syringe and change the needle.
4 The doctor expels all air bubbles from the syringe and most of the heparin, leaving only a very small volume to prevent the blood from clotting. He swabs the area and withdraws the blood. (Figure **173**)
5 Apply firm pressure to the puncture site for at least five minutes to prevent haematoma formation.
6 The needle on the syringe is replaced with a cap. The syringe is labelled, put into a receiver, covered with ice and sent to the laboratory immediately with the completed request card.
7 Apply an adhesive wound dressing to the puncture site.

**172**

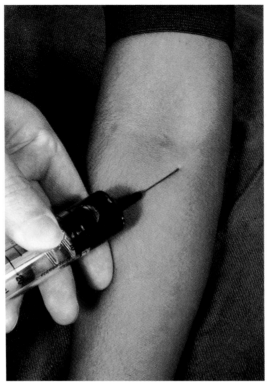

**173**

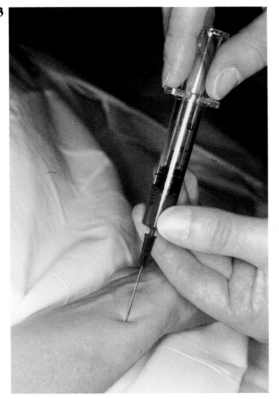

# 53 Intravenous injection

## Use
To give a drug directly into a vein.

## Equipment
a) Syringe, large enough for the volume of drug to be given.
b) Two sterile needles, 23 gauge.
c) Alcohol-impregnated swabs.
d) The prescribed drug, together with the correct fluid in which to dissolve it if necessary, and the relevant prescription sheet.
e) Tourniquet.
f) Elastic adhesive wound dressing.

## Procedure
1 Explain the procedure to the patient. Position him lying down in comfort and expose his arm, from above the elbow to the hand.
2 Draw up the correct dose of the drug, dissolving it in fluid if necessary. Change the needle on the syringe and expel any air from the syringe.
3 A doctor and a qualified nurse check that the drug and the dose are correct according to the prescription sheet.
4 Apply the tourniquet above the elbow and ask the patient to open and close his fist a few times, to engorge the veins with blood.
5 The doctor swabs the arm, introduces the needle and withdraws a small volume of blood to ensure that the needle is in a vein (Figure **174**). He removes the tourniquet and injects the drug, usually slowly. He places a swab over the injection site and removes the needle from the arm.
6 Apply pressure over the puncture site until bleeding stops, then apply an adhesive wound dressing.
7 Ensure that the prescription sheet is signed, to show that the drug has been given. Record the time.
*N.B.* Intravenous injections can also be given via an indwelling cannula or an intravenous infusion set.

# 54 Intracardiac injection

## Use
To give a drug directly into the heart, during resuscitation following a cardiac arrest.

## Equipment
a) Syringe, large enough for the volume of drug to be given.
b) Long sterile spinal needle.
c) Sterile needle, 23 gauge.
d) Alcohol-impregnated swab
e) The prescribed drug.

## Procedure
1 Draw up the correct dose of the drug and expel any air from the syringe.
2 A doctor and a qualified nurse check that the drug and the dose are correct.
3 The doctor swabs the chest in the area where he will inject the drug (about the fourth intercostal space to the left of the sternum). He introduces the spinal needle (Figures **175,176**) and removes the stylet. He connects the syringe to the needle, withdraws blood to check that the needle is in the heart, injects the drug and withdraws the needle.
4 Ensure that, when the opportunity arises, the doctor prescribes the drug in writing and records that he has given it.

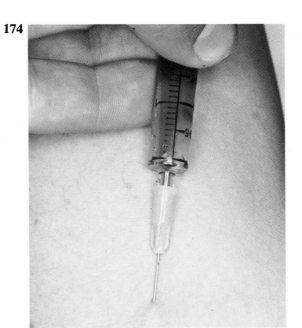

**174**

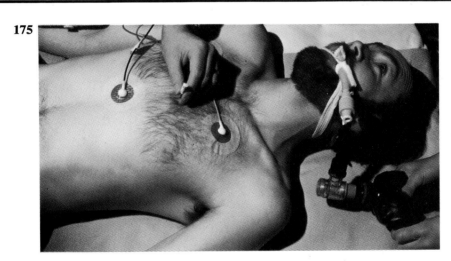

**175**

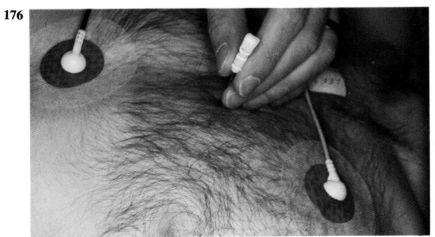

**176**

# 55 Intravenous infusion

## Uses
1 To give fluids directly into the circulation.
2 To provide ready access to the circulation in order to give drugs.

## Equipment
*a)* Drip stand.
*b)* Bag (or bottle) of the prescribed fluid.
*c)* Giving-set.
*d)* Razor.
*e)* Intravenous cannula.
*f)* Alcohol-impregnated swabs.
*g)* Tourniquet.
*h)* Elastic adhesive bandage, 7.5cm width.
*i)* Permeable adhesive tape, 1.25cm width.
*j)* Splint.
*k)* Cotton conforming bandage, 7.5cm width.
*l)* Fluid balance chart.

## Procedure
1 Explain the procedure to the patient. Position him lying down in comfort.
2 Check that the patient is not allergic to elastic adhesive bandage; if so, substitute a non-allergenic tape.
3 Cut a 'T' shape at the centre of the elastic adhesive bandage. (Figure **177**)
4 Check the fluid with the doctor. Hang the bag of fluid on the drip stand. Remove the protective cover from the fluid bag and also from the giving-set.
5 Push the regulator on the giving-set along the tubing to a point below the chambers.
6 Insert the giving-set into the bag of fluid and gently squeeze the bag to fill the chambers about one-third full. (Figure **178**)
7 Release the regulator to allow fluid to run through the tubing to expel all air-bubbles. Then turn off the fluid.
8 *Insertion of the intravenous cannula:*
    A Expose the selected area (usually the forearm) and shave any excess hair.
    B Apply the tourniquet above the elbow and ask the patient to open and close his fist a few times, to engorge the veins with blood.
    C The doctor swabs the area, introduces the cannula (Figures **179,180**) and removes the tourniquet.
    D If the doctor wishes to take a specimen of blood at this stage, hand him the correct syringe and ensure the required bottles and laboratory request forms are readily available (see page 96).

9 The doctor connects the giving-set to the cannula, releases the regulator and ensures that the fluid is flowing satisfactorily into the vein.
10 Secure the cannula with permeable adhesive tape and then with the elastic adhesive bandage. (Figures **181,182**)
11 Secure the giving-set with tape and/or cotton conforming bandage. (Figure **183**)
12 A splint may be applied if necessary.
13 Record the time the infusion commenced on the fluid balance chart. The doctor will prescribe a fluid regime.

## Advice to patients
Move the limb as carefully as possible, to avoid dislodging the cannula.

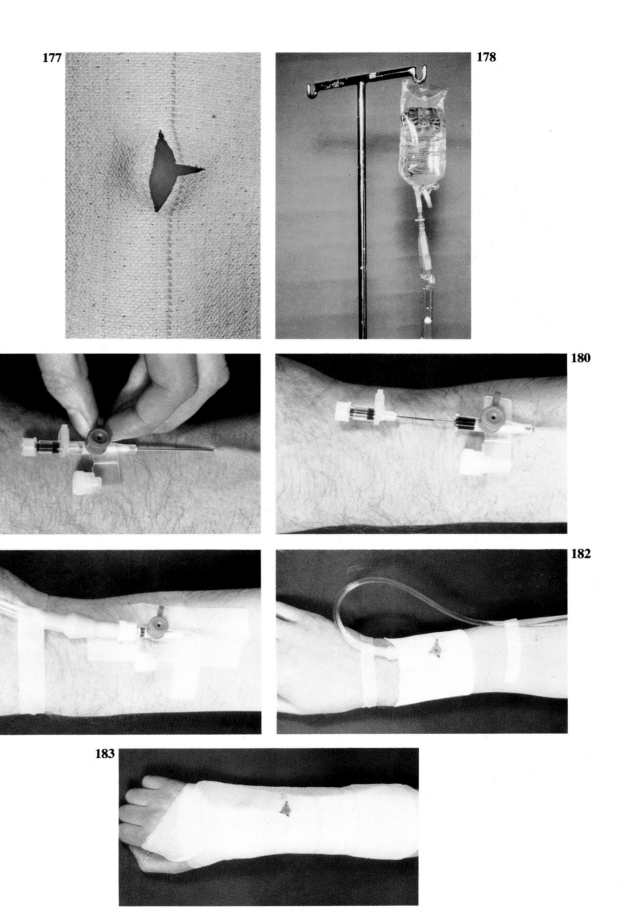

# 56 Cut-down for intravenous infusion

## Use
To set up an intravenous infusion when it is impossible to gain access to a vein in the usual way, usually because the patient is severely shocked.

## Equipment
a) Sterile intravenous cut-down set, comprising:
    Scalpel handle
    Fine toothed forceps
    Fine non-toothed forceps
    Two mosquito artery forceps
    Small straight pointed scissors
    Hook
    Aneurysm needle
    Small skin-retractor
    Needle holder
    Paper towels
    Gauze
    Cotton wool balls
    Tray

b) Two scalpel blades.
c) Cleansing solution.
d) Skin suture material.
e) Absorbable suture material.
f) 5ml syringe.
g) 5ml ampoule of 1% plain lignocaine.
h) Sterile needle, 23 gauge.
i) Surgeon's gloves.
j) Masks.
k) Equipment for intravenous infusion (see page 100).

## Procedure
N.B. Aseptic technique must be used.
1 Explain the procedure to the patient. Position him lying down in comfort.
2 Check that the patient is not allergic to elastic adhesive bandage; if so, substitute a non-allergenic tape.
3 Check the fluid with the doctor. Hang the bag of fluid on the drip stand. Remove the protective cover from the fluid bag and from the giving-set.
4 Push the regulator on the giving-set along the tubing to a point below the chambers.
5 Insert the giving-set into the bag of fluid and gently squeeze the bag to fill the chambers about one-third full.
6 Release the regulator to allow fluid to run through the tubing to expel all air-bubbles. Then turn off the fluid.
7 Expose the selected area and shave any excess hair.
8 The doctor prepares the sterile field and draws up and checks the lignocaine, swabs the area and injects the lignocaine to provide local anaesthesia.

9 The doctor incises the skin and dissects the tissues to expose the vein (Figure 184). He puts two lengths of absorbable suture material around the vein and ties the one furthest from the heart (Figure 185). He opens the vein, introduces the cannula, and ties it into the vein with the other length of absorbable suture material (Figure 186). He connects the giving-set to the cannula and asks the nurse to release the regulator to ensure that the fluid flows satisfactorily into the vein. He closes the wound with suture material and uses a skin suture to secure the cannula to the skin. (Figure 187)
10 If the doctor wishes to take a specimen of blood at this stage, hand him the correct syringe and ensure the required bottles and laboratory request cards are readily available (see page 96).
11 Secure the cannula and giving-set with permeable adhesive tape and then with the elastic adhesive bandage and/or cotton conforming bandage.
12 A splint may be applied if necessary.
13 Record the time the infusion commenced on the fluid balance chart. The doctor will prescribe a fluid regime.

## Advice to patients
Move the limb as carefully as possible, to avoid dislodging the cannula.

**184**

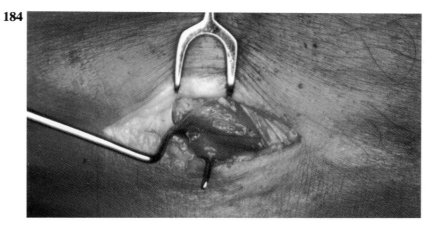

**185**

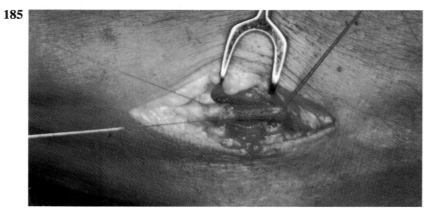

**186**

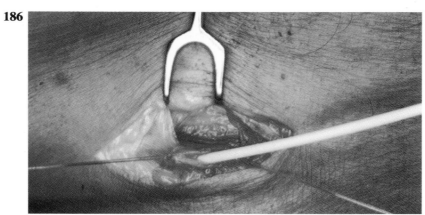

**187**

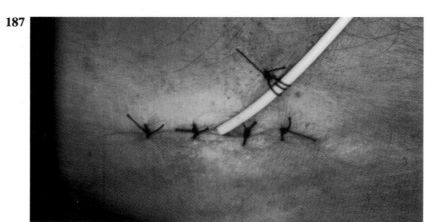

# 57 Incision and drainage

## Use
To release pus from an infected area.

## Equipment
a) Sterile suture set, comprising:
  Scalpel handle
  Toothed forceps
  Non-toothed forceps
  Spencer-Wells forceps
  Needle holder
  Sinus forceps
  Scissors
  Paper towels
  Gauze
  Cotton wool balls
  Tray
b) Scalpel blade.
c) Volkmann's spoon.
d) Ribbon gauze.
e) Cleansing solution.
f) Topical antiseptic solution (Eusol or proflavine cream).
g) Sterile towels.
h) Surgeon's gloves.
i) Bacteriology swab.
j) Laboratory request card.

## Procedure
N.B. General or local anaesthesia is required, as prescribed by the doctor.
  Aseptic technique must be used.
1 Explain the procedure to the patient. Position him lying down in comfort.
2 Test the patient's urine for sugar.
3 Expose the affected area. (Figure **188**)
4 The doctor cleans the area, positions the towels and incises the lesion, releasing the pus. (Figure **189**)
5 A bacteriology swab is taken. (Figure **190**)
6 The doctor may curette the lesion with a Volkmann's spoon, to break down pockets of infection. The area is cleaned. (Figure **191**)
7 The ribbon gauze is soaked in topical antiseptic solution and used to pack the wound (see page 72). (Figure **192**)
8 The wound is covered with gauze and a dry dressing is applied (see page 54).
9 Label the bacteriology swab, complete the laboratory request card and send both to the laboratory.

## Advice to patients
Keep the dressing clean and dry.
If there is excessive leaking through the dressing, return to hospital.
Exercise, rest or elevate the affected area, according to the doctor's instructions.

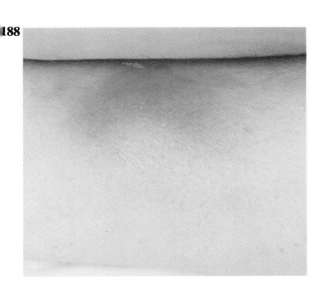

188

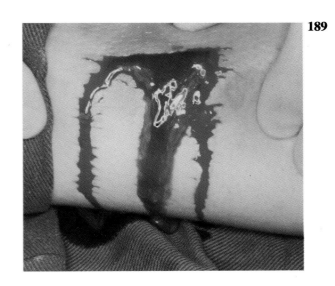

189

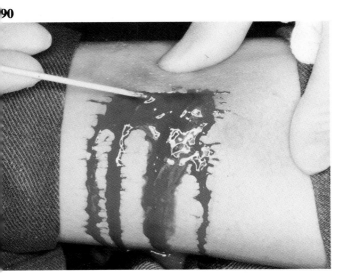

90

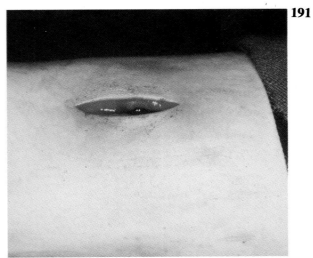

191

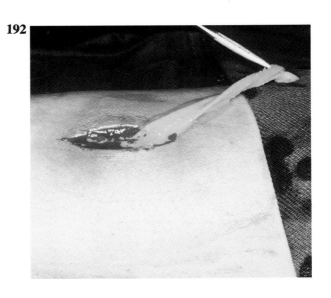

192

# 58 Suturing

## Use
To close a wound.

## Equipment
*a)* Sterile suture set, comprising:
      Scalpel handle
      Toothed forceps
      Non-toothed forceps
      Spencer-Wells forceps
      Needle holder
      Sinus forceps
      Scissors
      Paper towels
      Gauze
      Cotton wool balls
      Tray
*b)* Cleansing solution.
*c)* Suture material(s).
*d)* Scalpel blade(s). ⎤
*e)* Surgeon's gloves. ⊢— *(optional)*
*f)* Masks. ⎦

## Procedure
*N.B.* General or local anaesthesia may be required, as
    prescribed by the doctor.
    Ensure that the patient is adequately immunised
    against tetanus.
    Aseptic technique must be used.
1 Explain the procedure to the patient. Position him
  lying down in comfort.
2 Expose the affected area; wound toilet will have been
  performed already (see page 70). (Figure **193**)
3 The doctor may excise the wound edges if they are
  dirty or irregular.
4 The doctor sutures the wound; the nurse swabs away
  any blood with gauze. (Figures **194-196**)
5 Cut the sutures about 0.5cm from the knot, unless the
  doctor asks otherwise. (Figures **197,198**)
6 Reassure the patient as the procedure continues.
7 Apply the appropriate dressing.

## Advice to patients
Keep the dressing clean and dry.
If the wound becomes red or painful or leaks pus, return
to hospital.
Exercise, rest or elevate the affected area, according to
the doctor's instructions.

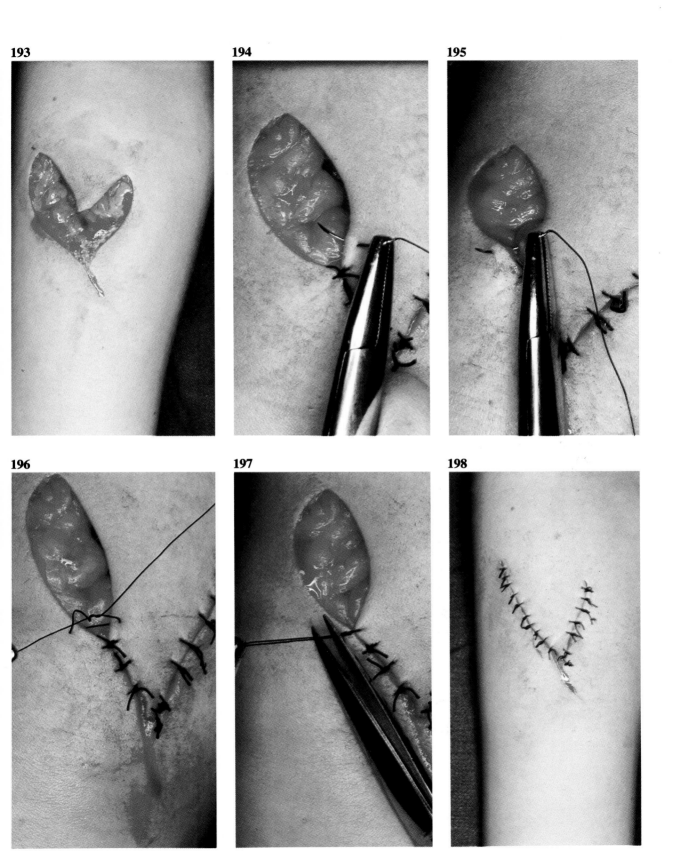

# 59 Knee aspiration

## Use
To remove fluid from a knee joint.

## Equipment
a) Sterile knee aspiration set, comprising:
- Surgeon's gown
- Measuring jug
- Towels
- Swab holder
- Receiver
- Gauze
- Cotton wool balls
- Tray

b) Cleansing solution.
c) Weak iodine solution.
d) 5ml syringe.
e) 5ml ampoule of 1% plain lignocaine.
f) Sterile needle, 25 gauge.
g) Surgeon's gloves.
h) Masks.
i) 20ml syringe.
j) Sterile needle, 19 gauge.
k) Sterile specimen pot.
l) Laboratory request card.
m) Clear plastic dressing spray.

## Procedure
*N.B.* Aseptic technique must be used.

1 Explain the procedure to the patient. Position him lying down in comfort with his leg exposed.
2 The doctor cleans the area of the knee with cleansing solution followed by weak iodine solution and positions the sterile towels. He draws up the lignocaine and injects it at the site of aspiration, which is usually in the superolateral area of the knee. (Figure **199**)
3 The doctor uses the 20ml syringe and the 19 gauge needle to aspirate the fluid from the knee joint. (Figure **200**)
4 The appearance and volume of the aspirated fluid are recorded.
5 A specimen is taken in a sterile pot, which is labelled and sent to the laboratory with a completed request card.
6 Apply the plastic dressing spray and a dry dressing (see page 54) to the site of aspiration.
7 Apply a Robert Jones pressure bandage (see page 46) or a wool and crepe bandage (see page 18), according to the doctor's instructions.

## Advice to patients
Use the walking aid provided (see page 24).
Keep the dressing dry.
Exercise the ankle and quadriceps muscle as follows: hold the foot at right angles and tighten the muscle at the front of the thigh; raise the straightened leg for five seconds and lower it slowly; rotate the ankle clockwise and anti-clockwise. Repeat these exercises for five minutes every hour, during the day.
If the foot becomes discoloured, numb or excessively swollen, return to hospital.
Follow the doctor's instructions regarding elevation of the leg, weight-bearing and mobility.

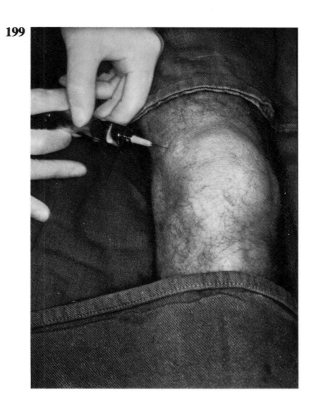

199

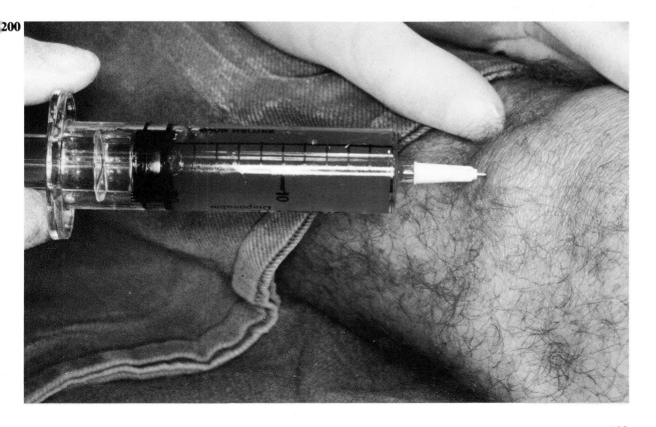

200

# 60 Insertion of a Steinmann's pin

## Uses
1 To apply skeletal traction, via the upper tibia, to a fractured shaft of femur.
2 To apply skeletal traction, via the calcaneus, to a fractured shaft of tibia.
3 To apply external fixation.

## Equipment
*a)* Sterile Steinmann's pin set, comprising:
    Steinmann's pins, of various sizes
    Stirrups, of various sizes
    Universal handle and key
    Two pin-guards
    Sponge holder
    Scissors
    Scalpel handle
    Spencer-Wells forceps
    Orthopaedic hammer
    Gallipot
    Paper towels
    Gauze
    Non-adherent absorbent dressing
    Tray

*b)* Cleansing solution.
*c)* Weak iodine solution.
*d)* 10ml syringe.
*e)* 10ml ampoule of 1% plain lignocaine.
*f)* Sterile needle, 21 gauge.
*g)* Surgeon's gown.
*h)* Surgeon's gloves.
*i)* Masks.
*j)* Sterile towels.
*k)* Scalpel blade.
*l)* Clear plastic dressing spray.
*m)* Permeable adhesive tape.

## Procedure
*N.B.* Two nurses are required.
    Aseptic technique must be used.
1 Explain the procedure to the patient. Position him lying down in comfort with his leg exposed.
2 The doctor cleans the area with cleansing solution followed by weak iodine solution and positions the sterile towels (Figure **201**). He draws up the lignocaine and injects about 5ml in the area where the pin is to be introduced, infiltrating the skin and tissues to the bone.
3 The doctor makes a small incision in the skin with the scalpel and introduces the pin through this. He pushes the pin, using the universal handle, through the tissues and on through the bone. (Figure **202**)
4 When the pin reaches the opposite cortex of the bone, the doctor infiltrates about 5ml of lignocaine into the skin and tissues to the bone, in the area from which he expects the pin to emerge. (Figure **203**)

5 The doctor pushes the pin through the opposite cortex, makes a small cut in the skin where the pin will emerge and pushes the pin through. The pin now passes right through the leg. (Figure **204**)
6 Apply the plastic dressing spray around the sites of entry and exit of the pin. Non-adherent absorbent dressing is placed over the areas, to protect the sites, and is secured with permeable adhesive tape. (Figure **205**)
7 A stirrup is fixed to the pin and pin-guards are applied to the two ends of the pin. (Figure **206**)
8 The patient is made comfortable and taken to the ward, where traction will be applied.

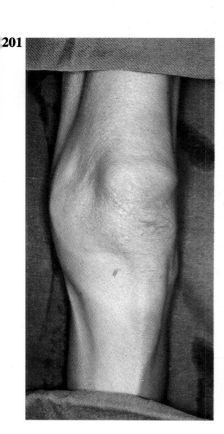

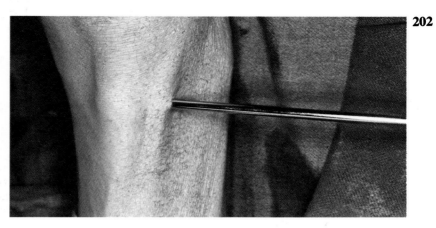

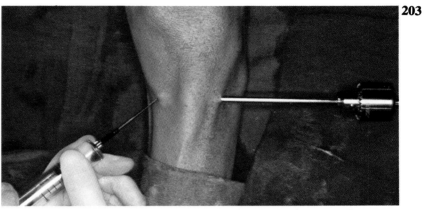

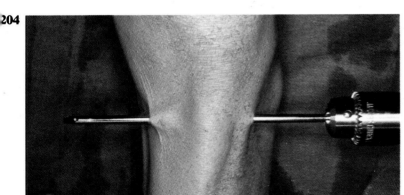

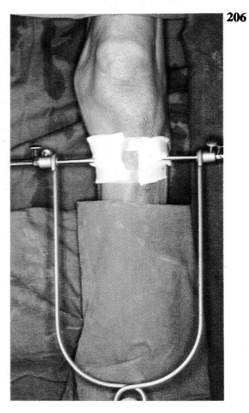

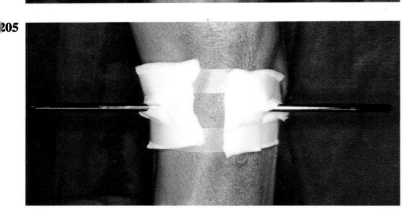

# 61 Chest intubation

## Uses
1 To allow air (that is, a pneumothorax) to escape from the pleural cavity.
2 To allow other fluids (usually blood, a haemothorax, in the Accident and Emergency Department) to drain from the pleural cavity.

## Equipment
a) Sterile thoracic pack, comprising:
>  Two sponge-holding forceps
>  Scalpel handle
>  Spencer-Wells forceps
>  Toothed forceps
>  Non-toothed forceps
>  Sinus forceps
>  Needle holder
>  Scissors
>  Two towel-clips
>  Two gate clamps
>  Paper towels
>  Gauze
>  Cotton wool balls
>  Tray

b) Sterile chest-bottle and tubing set, comprising:
>  Chest bottle
>  Rubber bung, with a short piece and a long piece of right-angled glass tubing through it
>  Rubber tubing
>  Sterile towels
>  Connections

c) Cleansing solution.
d) 10ml syringe.
e) 10ml ampoule of 1% lignocaine.
f) Sterile needle, 21 gauge.
g) Surgeon's gloves.
h) Masks.
i) Sterile towels.
j) Scalpel blade(s).
k) Suture material.
l) Two heavy clamps.
m) Trocar-catheter, of suitable length and diameter.
n) Indelible pen.
o) One litre of sterile distilled water and measuring jug.
p) Elastic adhesive tape, 7.5cm width.
q) Plastic adhesive strapping, 7.5cm width.
r) Non-adherent absorbent dressing, 10cm × 10cm.
s) Absorbent dressing pad.

## Procedure
N.B. Aseptic technique must be used.
1 Explain the procedure to the patient. Position him in comfort on a trolley, sitting upright if possible. Undress the patient to the waist.
2 Measure one litre of sterile water and pour into the chest bottle, marking the water level on the bottle with elastic adhesive tape; write the volume of water used on the tape.
3 Put the bung into the bottle and tape in place with elastic adhesive tape around the neck of the bottle. The lower end of the long piece of glass tubing is below the water level; the short piece is well above the water.
4 The doctor may mark the site selected for intubation with an indelible pen: this site is usually the second intercostal space just outside the midclavicular line (for air) or the eighth intercostal space in the midaxillary line (for fluid). (Figure **207**)
5 The doctor cleans the area with cleansing solution and positions the sterile towels. He injects lignocaine into the selected site, infiltrating to the pleura.
6 The doctor may put a pursestring suture around the selected site; this suture will be tied when the drain is eventually removed. (Figure **208**)
7 A transverse incision is made just above the upper border of the rib and down to the pleura. Spencer-Wells forceps may be used to open up the tissues.
8 The doctor introduces the trocar-catheter into the pleural cavity. Reassure the patient, since this procedure can be uncomfortable. (Figure **209**)
9 The doctor removes the trocar and immediately clamps the catheter. (Figure **210**)
10 The catheter is connected to the underwater seal with rubber tubing and connections.
11 The chest bottle is placed on the floor.
12 The doctor removes the clamp from the catheter and checks that the water-level swings when the patient coughs: this indicates that the catheter is positioned correctly.
13 The catheter is anchored securely with one or two sutures. (Figure **211**)
14 A non-adherent dressing and an absorbent dressing pad are positioned around the catheter where it emerges from the chest wall and secured with plastic adhesive strapping. (Figure **212**)
15 A chest X-ray is taken to check that the catheter is positioned correctly.
16 When transporting the patient, the rubber tubing must be clamped in two places with heavy clamps, to ensure that water does not enter the chest.

N.B. Ensure that the bottle is always well below the level of the chest. (Figure **213**)

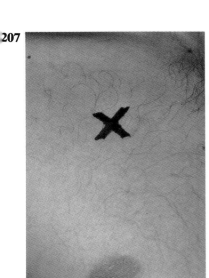

**207**

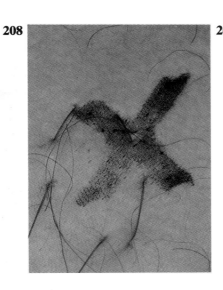

**208**

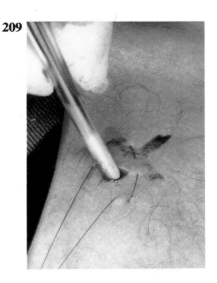

**209**

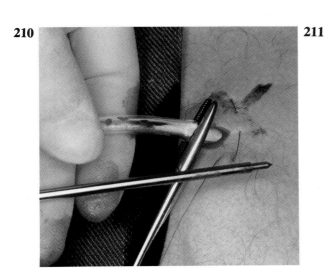

**210**

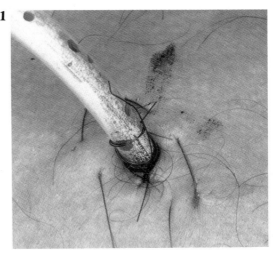

**211**

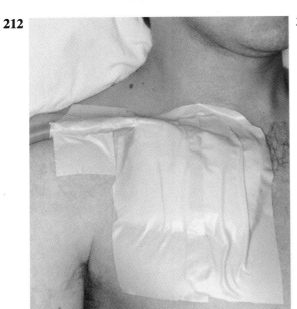

**212**

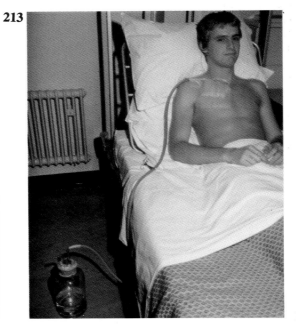

**213**

# 62 Removal of a foreign body: (A) from the eye

## Equipment
a) Cotton bud.
b) Sterile needle, 23 gauge.
c) Amethocaine 1% eye drops.
d) Fluorescein 2% eye drops.
e) Sodium chloride 0.9% eye drops.
f) Antibiotic eye drops and/or ointment.
g) Eye pad.
h) Permeable adhesive tape.
i) Torch.
j) Magnifying loupe, magnifying spectacles or slit-lamp microscope.
N.B. Good lighting is essential.

## Procedure
1 Explain the procedure to the patient. Remove any contact lenses.
2 The patient's head must be kept completely still. Usually the patient is seated in a special eye-chair, with his head firmly supported on the headrest. Alternatively, he may lie on a trolley.
3 The doctor examines the eye and locates the foreign body. (Figure **214**)
4 Sometimes it is possible to remove the foreign body by irrigation (see page 128) or with a cotton bud. If not, the doctor puts two or three drops of amethocaine into the eye to provide local anaesthesia: this stings briefly.
5 The patient fixes his gaze on a stationary object and the foreign body is picked out of the cornea, using a sterile needle. (Figure **215**)
6 If the foreign body contains iron, it may leave a rust-ring which the doctor can scrape off carefully with a needle.
7 A few drops of fluorescein can be put into the eye: this will show up any scratches on the cornea as green fluorescent stains when light is shone obliquely across the eye.
8 To examine under the upper eyelid, ask the patient to look down and gently press the cotton bud along the upper margin of the lid; then ask the patient to open both eyes and evert the upper eyelid by gently pulling the lashes downwards, then forwards, then upwards. A foreign body under the lid can then be removed. (Figure **216**)
9 Rinse the eye with sodium chloride.
10 If a corneal ulcer or abrasion remains, antibiotic drops and/or ointment will be prescribed by the doctor.
11 If amethocaine has been used, an eye pad is placed over the closed eye and secured with one or two pieces of permeable adhesive tape, applied from the forehead to the cheek. (Figure **217**)

## Advice to patients
The eye pad must be worn for at least six hours.
Do not drive while wearing the eye pad; do not smoke as it is highly inflammable.
Use antibiotic eye drops and/or ointment as directed: pull down the lower lid and lightly smear the ointment along it. (Figure **218**)

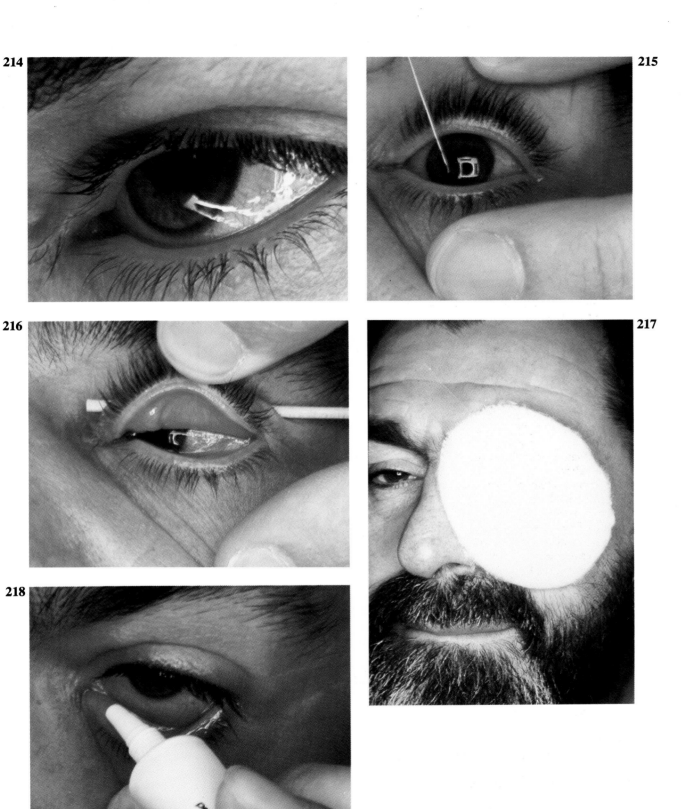

# 63 Removal of a foreign body: (B) from the ear

## Equipment
a) Auriscope.
b) Aural specula, of various sizes.
c) Tilley's nasal dressing forceps.
d) Strabismus hook.
e) Blunt right-angled probe.
f) Light source. Good lighting (for example, a headlight or a mirror with reflected light) is essential.

## Procedure
1 Explain the procedure to the patient.
2 The patient's head must be kept completely still. A child may require general anaesthesia or sedation and/or may need to be held firmly in a blanket. The patient should be positioned in comfort, either sitting in a chair with a headrest or lying on a trolley.
3 The doctor uses the auriscope and aural specula to locate the foreign body and assess its size, shape and consistency. It is essential that the foreign body is not pushed further into the ear and that the ear-drum is not damaged. (Figure **219**)

4 If the doctor feels it is safe to do so, he removes the foreign body, using forceps or strabismus hook or probe.
5 If the doctor feels it is unsafe to remove the foreign body, he refers the patient to an E.N.T. surgeon, who can remove it under general anaesthesia or with other instruments or suction.
6 It is inadvisable to attempt to syringe out a foreign body in the Accident and Emergency Department.
7 After removal of the foreign body, the doctor examines the ear to check that no foreign body remains and that the external auditory meatus and the ear-drum are not damaged.

# 64 Removal of a foreign body: (C) from the nose

## Equipment
a) Nasal specula, of various sizes.
b) Tilley's nasal dressing forceps.
c) Strabismus hook.
d) Blunt right-angled probe.
e) Light source. Good lighting (for example, a headlight or a mirror with reflected light) is essential.

## Procedure
1 Explain the procedure to the patient.
2 The patient's head must be kept completely still. A child may require general anaesthesia or sedation and/or may need to be held firmly in a blanket. The patient should be positioned in comfort, either sitting in a chair with a headrest or lying on a trolley in a head-up position.
3 The doctor uses a nasal speculum to locate the foreign body and assess its size, shape and consistency. It is essential that the foreign body is not pushed further up the nose. (Figure **220**)
4 The doctor may try to milk out the foreign body by pressure from above it. He may occlude the non-blocked nostril and ask the patient to blow the nose; if he sees the object, he applies pressure above it, to prevent it from slipping back into the nose.

5 If the above methods are unsuccessful and the doctor feels it is safe to do so, he removes the foreign body using forceps or strabismus hook or probe; he occludes the nostril above the foreign body as it is withdrawn, to prevent it from slipping back into the nose.
6 If the doctor feels it is unsafe to remove the foreign body, he refers the patient to an E.N.T. surgeon, who can remove it under general anaesthesia or with other instruments or suction.
7 After removal of the foreign body, the doctor examines the nose to check that no foreign body remains and that no damage has been caused.

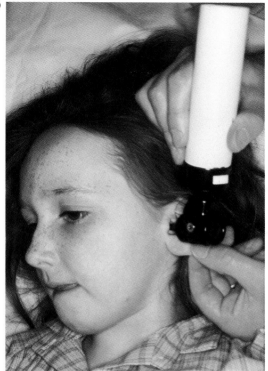

**219**

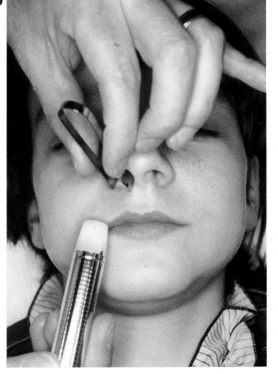

**220**

# 65 Pre- and postoperative care for general anaesthesia

## Use
To prepare a patient for a general anaesthetic and to ensure safe recovery afterwards.

## Equipment

### A PRE-OPERATIVE
a) Patient's gown and theatre cap.
b) Permeable adhesive tape.
c) Denture pot.
d) Name band.
e) Consent form.
f) Razor.
g) Patient's notes and X-rays.

### B POSTOPERATIVE
a) Oxygen.
b) Suction.
c) Airways.

## Procedure

### A PRE-OPERATIVE

1 Ideally, the patient should not eat or drink for at least four hours before a general anaesthetic. If the operation is very urgent, the anaesthetist may pass an endotracheal tube or empty the stomach with a gastric tube.
2 Explain the procedure to the patient.
3 The anaesthetist may prescribe certain drugs (e.g. atropine or diazepam) to be given shortly before the anaesthetic.
4 The anaesthetist may request an E.C.G. (see page 144), a chest X-ray or certain blood tests before the anaesthetic.
5 Dress the patient in a gown and theatre cap.
6 Remove all jewellery and nail-polish. Store jewellery with the patient's property. Rings which cannot be removed are covered completely with permeable adhesive tape.
7 Place any dentures in a labelled denture pot. Ask the patient if he has any crowns or bridges and advise the anaesthetist accordingly. Remove any contact lenses; store with the patient's property.
8 Place a name band around the patient's wrist: check that the details correspond with those on the case notes.
9 Record the patient's routine observations (temperature, pulse, blood pressure, respiratory rate): these are used as a base-line for subsequent observations.
10 Test the patient's urine and record the result.
11 The doctor will obtain the patient's consent (parent's or guardian's for a minor) for operation: the nurse should check that the consent form has been signed and is with the case notes.
12 Wash and shave the area to be treated, if required.

### B POSTOPERATIVE

1 Ensure that the patient's airway passage is clear and that his breathing is satisfactory. Oxygen, suction and airways must be immediately available.
2 Nurse the patient on his side until he regains consciousness. (Figure 221)
3 Record the routine observations ¼-hourly until consciousness is regained, then ½-hourly until they are stable.
4 When the patient regains consciousness, reassure him and advise him to rest.
5 About one hour later, he may sit up and drink.
6 On discharge, the patient should be accompanied by a relative or friend.

## Advice to patients
Do not drive for at least 24 hours.

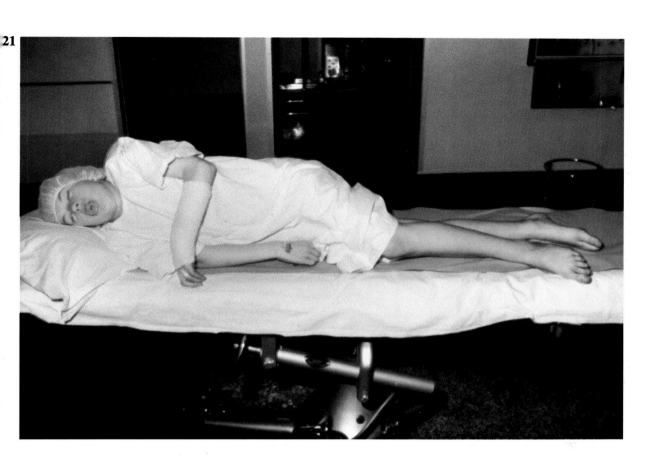

# 66 Brachial plexus (axillary) block

## Use
To provide anaesthesia of the forearm, wrist and hand for surgical procedures (for example, reduction of fractures or dislocations, tendon exploration and suture).

## Equipment
a) Two 20ml syringes.
b) Two sterile needles.
c) 1% prilocaine, 20-40ml for a 70kg adult.
d) A short length of small-bore extension tubing.
e) Tourniquet.
f) Alcohol-impregnated swabs.
g) Indwelling-needle, 21 gauge.
h) Permeable adhesive tape.
i) Cleansing solution.
j) Razor.
k) Sterile needle, 23 gauge.
l) Gauze.
m) Pillow to support the injured arm.
n) Resuscitation equipment.

## Procedure
1 Explain the procedure to the patient.
2 Remove all jewellery from the affected arm; store with the patient's property.
3 Dress the patient in a gown.
4 Record the patient's routine observations (temperature, pulse, blood pressure, respiratory rate).
5 Shave the axilla.
6 Position the patient in comfort on a trolley: the injured arm must be abducted to about 90° at the shoulder and the arm should be supported on a pillow with the elbow flexed, so that the hand lies a few inches from the head. (Figure 222)
7 The doctor draws up the required volume of prilocaine, attaches the extension tubing to the syringe and expels air from the tubing.
8 The doctor inserts an indwelling-needle into a vein in the uninjured arm and tapes it in place; this provides easy access to the circulation if required.
9 The doctor places the tourniquet around the injured arm about one-quarter of the way down the humerus, to keep the prilocaine in the axillary sheath. He swabs the axilla and introduces a 23 gauge needle just above the axillary artery, as high in the axilla as possible and pointing towards the apex of the axilla. The doctor feels a 'click' as the needle penetrates the axillary sheath and the patient may feel a shooting sensation down the arm. The needle is seen to pulsate.

10 The doctor connects the extension tubing to the needle in the axilla and injects the prilocaine, aspirating repeatedly to ensure the needle is not in a vessel (Figure 223). Having completed the injection, the doctor removes the needle from the axilla. The injured arm is brought down to the patient's side.
11 Record the time. The tourniquet is removed 20 minutes after the injection.
12 Surgery can begin about 30 minutes after the injection.
13 After surgery, remove the indwelling-needle from the uninjured arm.
14 Record the patient's observations.

## Advice to patients
Normal sensation may take up to 16 hours to return.

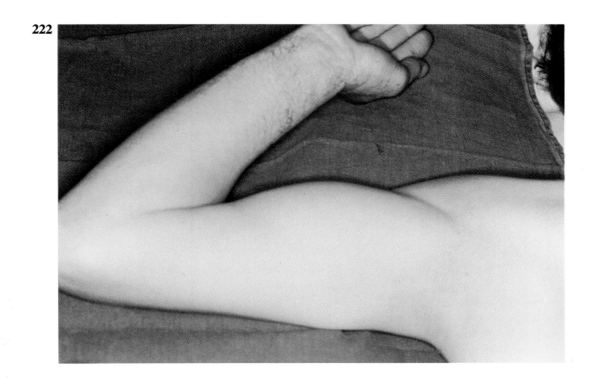

**222**

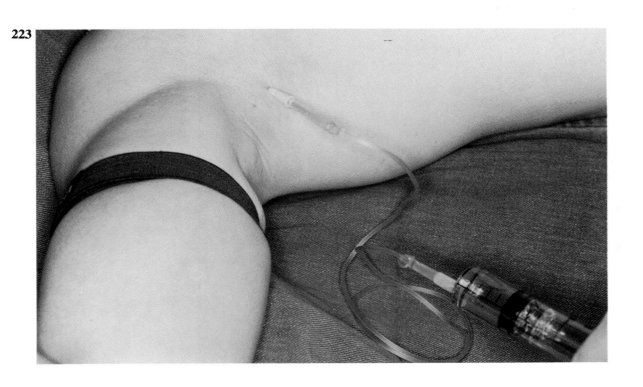

**223**

# 67 Bier's block (intravenous regional anaesthesia)

## Use
To provide anaesthesia of the forearm, wrist and hand for simple surgical procedures (for example, reduction of a Colles' fracture).

The method can be adapted for use in the lower leg.

## Equipment
a) Pneumatic cuff, with attached pressure gauge and equipment for controlling the pressure in the cuff. (An ordinary sphygmomanometer cuff is unsafe and must never be used.)
b) Surgical wool.
c) Two 20ml syringes.
d) Two sterile needles.
e) 0.5% prilocaine, 40ml for a 70kg adult.
f) Tourniquet.
g) Alcohol-impregnated swabs.
h) Two indwelling-needles, 21 gauge.
i) Permeable adhesive tape.
j) Gauze.
k) Resuscitation equipment.

## Procedure
1 Explain the procedure to the patient.
2 Record the patient's routine observations (temperature, pulse, blood pressure, respiratory rate) and weigh him.
3 Dress the patient in a gown and position him lying down in comfort.
4 Remove all jewellery; store with the patient's property.
5 Check the pneumatic cuff to ensure that pressure can be maintained and that there are no leaks.
6 The doctor draws up the required volume of prilocaine.
7 The doctor inserts an indwelling-needle into a vein in the uninjured arm, so that intravenous drugs can be given immediately if necessary.
8 Apply surgical wool around the upper arm (Figure 224) and place the pneumatic cuff over it, ensuring that the cuff is entirely underlaid with wool. Tie the cuff in position, so that it cannot become loose or unravel. (Figure 225)
9 The doctor inserts an indwelling-needle into a vein on the back of the hand and tapes it in position.
10 Ask the patient to raise the injured arm for about two minutes, helping him if necessary (Figure 226). This drains some of the blood from the veins. After two minutes, inflate the cuff to 250mm of mercury and lower the patient's arm.
11 Record the time.
12 The doctor injects the prilocaine into the indwelling-needle in the injured limb. (Figure 227)
13 The arm soon becomes blotchy in appearance. Surgery can begin about ten minutes after injection.
14 A nurse must continuously ensure that the pressure in the cuff remains at 250mm of mercury throughout the procedure.
15 After surgery, and at least thirty minutes after the injection of prilocaine, the doctor deflates the cuff gradually, over a couple of minutes. The cuff should not be inflated for more than 45 minutes.

16 The cuff, the surgical wool and the indwelling-needle are removed. The indwelling-needle is removed from the uninjured arm.
17 Record the patient's routine observations.
18 Keep the patient under observation for at least 45 minutes after deflation of the cuff.
19 Ensure the patient is accompanied by a relative or friend when discharged.

## Advice to patients
Normal sensation will return within about ten minutes of deflating the cuff. Occasionally there may be temporary minor side-effects soon after deflation (a metallic taste in the mouth, tingling in the hand or ringing in the ears).

N.B. There are recognised complications of intravenous regional anaesthesia (including convulsions, hypotension, respiratory depression and cardiac arrhythmias, which could lead to cardiac arrest). These can be avoided by using the above technique and taking the following precautions:

(a) The procedure should not be undertaken in patients with a history of epilepsy, cardiac disease, hypertension, sickle-cell disease, known hypersensitivity to local anaesthetic agents, porphyria, vascular disease of the limb or cellulitis of the limb.

(b) The patient should be starved for four hours before the procedure to minimise the risk of inhalation of stomach contents.

(c) The patient must be co-operative.

(d) One doctor is responsible solely for the anaesthesia and a second doctor is responsible for the surgery.

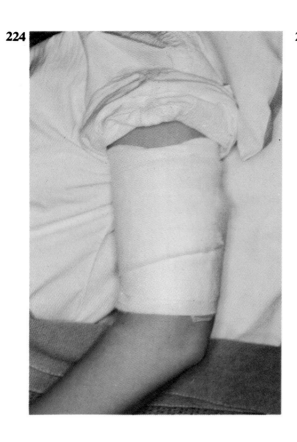

**224**

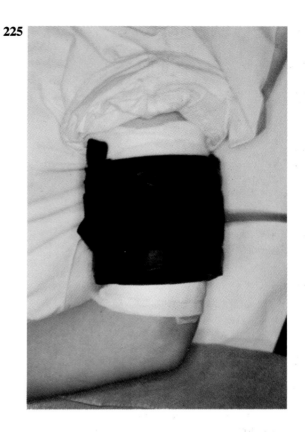

**225**

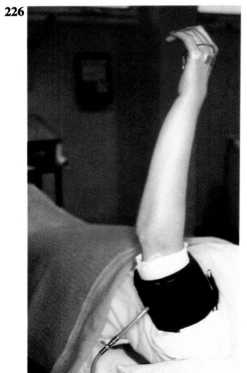

**226**

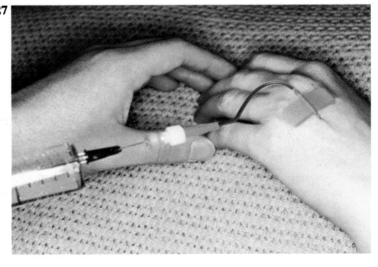

**227**

## 68 Ring block

### Use
To provide anaesthesia of a finger or toe for minor surgery.

### Equipment
a) 5ml syringe.
b) Sterile needle, 23 gauge.
c) 5ml ampoule of 1% plain lignocaine.
d) Alcohol-impregnated swab.

### Procedure
1 Explain the procedure to the patient.
2 Position the patient lying down in comfort and expose the affected hand or foot.
3 The doctor draws up the lignocaine and swabs the site for injection, at the base of the digit or in the web space.
4 The doctor injects some lignocaine next to the digital nerve (Figure **228**); then repeats the injection on the other side of the digit (Figure **229**).
5 The digit becomes anaesthetised within about three minutes; surgery then begins.

### Advice to patients
Normal sensation may take up to six hours to return.

## 69 Local anaesthesia by infiltration

### Use
To provide anaesthesia for minor surgery, for example exploring and suturing lacerations.

### Equipment
a) Syringe.
b) Sterile needle, 23 gauge.
c) Ampoules of plain lignocaine.
d) Alcohol-impregnated swabs.

### Procedure
1 Explain the procedure to the patient.
2 Position the patient lying down in comfort and expose the affected area.
3 The doctor draws up the lignocaine and swabs the area to be injected.
4 The doctor injects the lignocaine (Figures **230, 231**). Discomfort is reduced by piercing the skin as rarely as possible, by pushing the needle under the skin edge rather than through the skin surface and by injecting in different directions through one stab point if possible, by moving the needle under the skin.
5 The area becomes anaesthetised within about three minutes; surgery then begins.

### Advice to patients
Normal sensation may take up to eight hours to return.

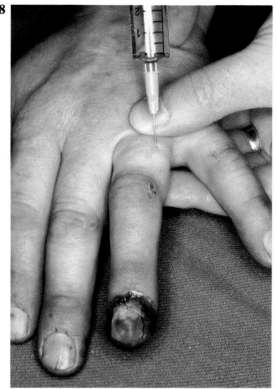

**228**

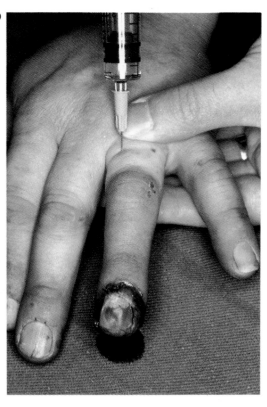

**229**

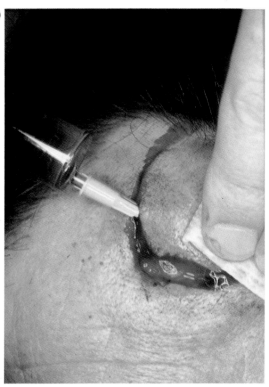

**230**

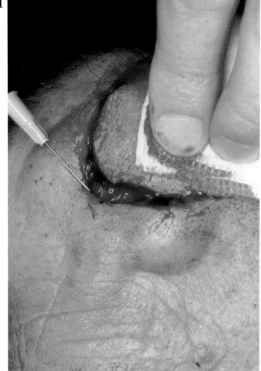

**231**

# 70 Anaesthesia with nitrous oxide/oxygen

## Use
To relieve pain and discomfort in a variety of procedures, for example removal of clothes from a fractured limb, splinting of fractures, reduction of certain fractures or dislocations, painful dressings.

## Equipment
*N.B.* Premixed nitrous oxide ($N_2O$) and oxygen ($O_2$) in the proportions of 50:50 in a single cylinder is available commercially; it supplies a constant predictable gas mixture which ensures adequate oxygenation while providing satisfactory pain relief.
*a)* Cylinder containing 50% nitrous oxide and 50% oxygen, with a demand-valve and mask attached for self-administration by the patient.
*b)* Trolley for transporting the cylinder.
*c)* Suction apparatus in case of vomiting.

## Procedure
1 Explain the procedure to the patient, stressing the pain relief available if he uses the equipment correctly.
2 Position the patient lying down in comfort.
3 Record the patient's routine observations (temperature, pulse, blood pressure, respiratory rate).
4 Instruct the patient in the self-administration of the gas, through a special demand-valve. He presses the mask to his face, covering the mouth and nose, and breathes in deeply. An air-tight seal between face and mask is important. A hissing sound is heard when the patient breathes in, if the apparatus is being used correctly. (Figure **232**)
5 Maximum pain relief develops in about two minutes, so painful procedures should be avoided for this time.
6 Encourage the patient throughout the procedure and supervise the correct use of the gas. Reassure him if he feels light-headed or restless.
7 After use, the mask should be cleaned with hot soapy water and then dried.

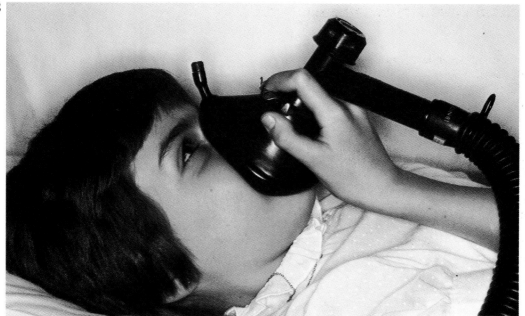

# 71 Eye irrigation

## Uses
1 To treat chemical burns of the eye (for example, by lime or cement).
2 To remove multiple small foreign bodies not embedded in the cornea (for example, sand or dust).

## Equipment
a) Plastic cape.
b) Receiver.
c) Water or normal saline solution.
d) Glass undine.
e) Litmus paper.
f) Amethocaine 1% eye drops.
g) Eye pad.
h) Permeable adhesive tape.
N.B. Good lighting is essential.

## Procedure
N.B. For chemical burns in particular, irrigation must be performed urgently, after the doctor has examined the eye.

1 Explain the procedure to the patient.
2 Position the patient in comfort in a special eye-chair, with his head firmly supported on the headrest. Alternatively, he may lie on a trolley.
3 Remove any contact lenses. Protect the patient's clothes with the plastic cape.
4 If the patient is unable to keep his eye open because of the irritation, put two or three drops of amethocaine into the eye to provide local anaesthesia: this will sting briefly.
5 Ask the patient to hold the receiver close to his jaw.
6 Tilt the patient's head slightly towards the affected side.
7 Fill the glass undine with water or normal saline solution.
8 Hold the patient's eyelids open with your free hand.
9 Allow some water or saline to flow over the cheek, close to the eye, so that the patient becomes used to the sensation.

10 Gradually moving towards the eye, let the water or saline flow freely across the surface of the eye, asking the patient to move the eyeball from side to side. (Figure **233**)
11 Refill the glass undine as necessary. The rate of flow can be controlled by placing your thumb over the inlet of the undine.
12 Litmus paper can be applied to the cornea to assess the pH when acid or alkaline substances have been in the eye.
13 If extensive irrigation is necessary, it may be preferable to use a 500ml bag of normal saline solution, an intravenous giving-set and a drip-stand. The patient lies on a trolley and the procedure is the same.
14 Any solid particles must be removed (see page 114).
15 If amethocaine has been used, an eye pad is placed over the closed eye and secured with one or two pieces of permeable adhesive tape, applied from the forehead to the cheek. (Figure **234**)

## Advice to patients
The eye pad must be worn for at least six hours.
Do not drive while wearing the eye pad; do not smoke as it is highly inflammable.
Use antibiotic eye drops and/or ointment as directed: pull down the lower lid and lightly smear the ointment along it. (Figure **235**)

**233**

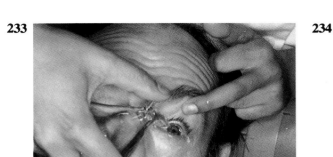

**234**

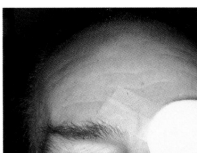

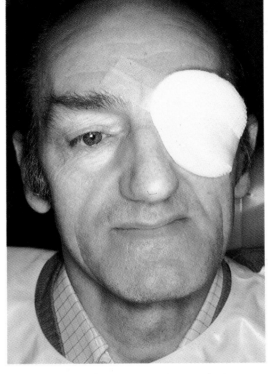

**235**

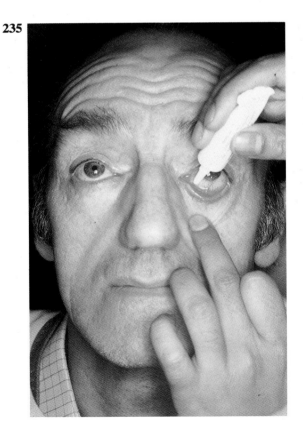

# 72 Nasal packing

## Use
To stop a nose-bleed.

## Equipment
a) Sterile dressing pack, comprising:
   Four pairs of non-toothed forceps
   Gallipot
   Paper towels
   Gauze
   Cotton wool balls
   Tray
b) Plastic cape.
c) Denture pot.
d) Receiver.
e) Tissues.
f) Bismuth, iodoform and paraffin paste (B.I.P.P.) impregnated ribbon gauze, or equivalent.
g) Nasal specula, of various sizes.
h) Tilley's nasal dressing forceps.
i) Permeable adhesive tape.
j) Scissors.

## Procedure
1 Explain the procedure to the patient.
2 Record the patient's routine observations (temperature, pulse, blood pressure, respiratory rate).
3 Place any dentures in a labelled denture pot.
4 Position the patient in comfort on a chair or trolley in a semi-recumbent position with his head well supported but tilted slightly backwards.
5 Protect the patient's clothes with the plastic cape.
6 Ensure a receiver is available for spitting out blood.
7 Place the B.I.P.P. gauze into the gallipot, using forceps.
8 Dilate the patient's nostril with a nasal speculum.
9 Ask the patient to breathe through his mouth.
10 Using Tilley's nasal dressing forceps, insert the end of the gauze along the floor of the nose for about 5cm.
11 Release the forceps and withdraw them. Pick up a loop of gauze about 5cm from the nostril: this loop and successive loops are packed on top of each other, filling the nasal cavity both from below upwards and from behind forwards. (Figure 236)
12 The packing must be applied firmly and fairly tightly. At the end of the procedure, the cut end of the gauze should be visible outside the nostril. Both nostrils are packed if necessary, according to the doctor's instructions. (Figure 237)
13 A piece of gauze is folded and taped under the nose to prevent the pack from being dislodged (Figure 238). Alternatively, a bolster can be made out of cotton tubular bandage and gauze, positioned under the nose and tied behind the patient's head. (Figure 239)
14 Provide a mouthwash.

## Advice to patients
Leave the pack in place for the instructed length of time (usually 48 hours).
If excessive bleeding appears through the pack, return to hospital.

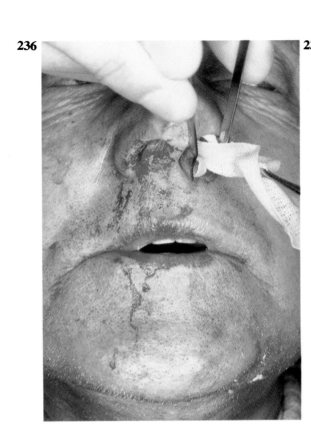

236

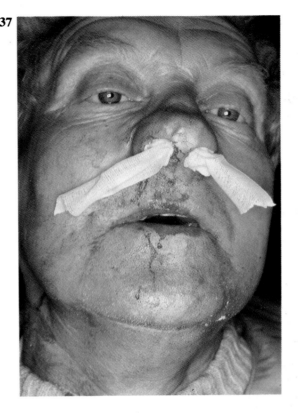

237

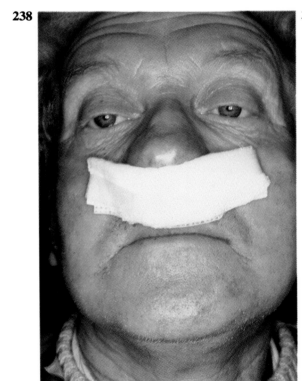

238

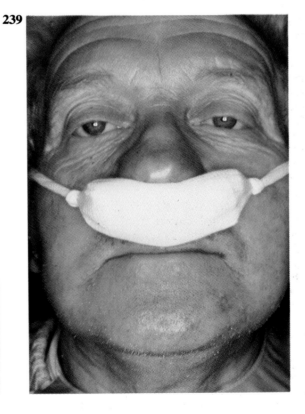

239

# 73 Catheterisation of the bladder: (A) male

## Uses
1 To relieve retention of urine.
2 To relieve incontinence of urine.
3 To measure urine output accurately.
4 To obtain a specimen of urine.
5 Following pelvic trauma.

## Equipment
a) Sterile catheterisation pack, comprising:
      One pair of non-toothed forceps
      Paper towel with central hole
      Nozzle for the lignocaine gel
      Receiver
      Gallipot
      Paper towels
      Gauze
      Cotton wool balls
b) Catheter.
c) Cleansing solution.
d) 15ml of sterile 2% lignocaine gel, with chlorhexidine.
e) Sterile water, syringe and sterile needle (if a balloon catheter is used).
f) Drainage bag.
g) Fluid chart.
h) Sterile specimen bottles and laboratory request forms.
i) Sterile gloves.
j) Sterile green towels.
k) Masks.

## Procedure
N.B. Aseptic technique must be used.
1 Explain the procedure to the patient.
2 Position the patient in comfort on his back with his legs slightly apart; expose the penis.
3 Position the sterile green towels or the paper towel with a central hole over the penis.
4 Retract the foreskin and clean the glans with cotton wool balls soaked in cleansing solution. (Figure 240)
5 Put the nozzle on the tube of lignocaine gel and squeeze the gel up the urethra, to anaesthetise and lubricate the urethra. (Figure 241)
6 Put a little lignocaine gel on the tip of the catheter to lubricate it.
7 Place the receiver between the patient's thighs.
8 After a few minutes, gently introduce the catheter into the penis and on into the bladder, using forceps and ensuring that you do not touch the catheter directly. (Figure 242)
9 When the catheter reaches the bladder, urine will flow through it; collect this in the receiver at first, until the drainage bag is connected.
10 If the catheter fails to pass easily, do not use force. A different type or size of catheter or an introducer may be required.
11 The volume of sterile water needed to fill the balloon of the catheter will be written on the catheter. Draw up this volume of sterile water into a syringe and use it to blow up the balloon.
12 Pull the catheter very gently to ensure it is retained in the bladder by the balloon.
13 Replace the foreskin.
14 If required, take specimens of urine in sterile specimen bottles, label them and send them to the laboratory with the completed request forms.
15 Connect the catheter to the drainage bag.
16 Test the urine and record the volume of urine drained on the fluid chart.
17 Ensure the patient is clean, dry and comfortable.

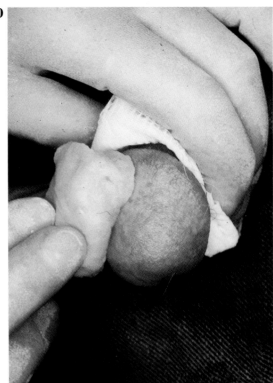

**240**

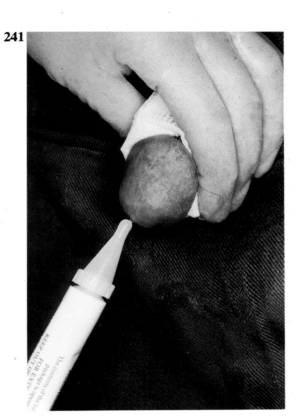

**241**

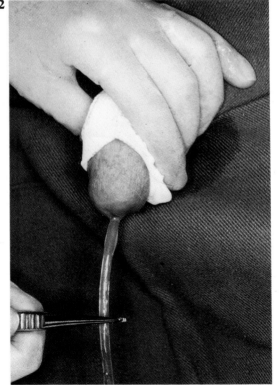

**242**

# 74 Catheterisation of the bladder: (B) female

## Uses
1 To relieve retention of urine.
2 To relieve incontinence of urine.
3 To measure urine output accurately.
4 To obtain a specimen of urine.
5 Following pelvic trauma.

## Equipment
a) Sterile catheterisation pack, comprising:
    One pair of non-toothed forceps
    Paper towel with central hole
    Receiver
    Gallipot
    Paper towels
    Gauze
    Cotton wool balls
b) Catheter.
c) Cleansing solution.
d) Sterile water, syringe and sterile needle (if a balloon catheter is used).
e) Drainage bag.
f) Fluid chart.
g) Sterile specimen bottles and laboratory request forms.
h) Sterile gloves.
i) Sterile green towels.
j) Masks.

## Procedure
N.B. Aseptic technique must be used.
1 Explain the procedure to the patient.
2 Position the patient in comfort on her back with her heels together and her knees apart, exposing the vulva.
3 Position the sterile green towels or the paper towel with a central hole over the vulva.
4 Separate the labia majora and clean the labia with cotton wool balls soaked in cleansing solution. Hold the swab with forceps if preferred and use each swab only once. Always swab from front to rear to reduce the chance of infection. Swab the labia majora first, then the labia minora and lastly the central area. (Figure **243**)
5 Place the receiver between the patient's thighs.
6 Gently introduce the catheter into the urethra and on into the bladder, using forceps and ensuring that you do not touch the catheter directly. (Figure **244**)
7 When the catheter reaches the bladder, urine will flow through it; collect this in the receiver at first, until the drainage bag is connected.
8 If the catheter fails to pass easily, do not use force. A different type or size of catheter or an introducer may be required.
9 The volume of sterile water needed to fill the balloon of the catheter will be written on the catheter. Draw up this volume of sterile water into a syringe and use it to blow up the balloon.
10 Pull the catheter very gently to ensure it is retained in the bladder by the balloon.
11 If required, take specimens of urine in sterile specimen bottles, label them and send them to the laboratory with the completed request forms.
12 Connect the catheter to the drainage bag.
13 Test the urine and record the volume of urine drained on the fluid chart.
14 Ensure the patient is clean, dry and comfortable.

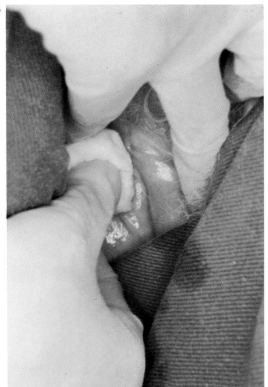

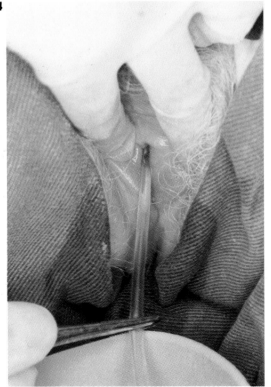

# 75  Removal of rings

## Use
To remove a ring from a finger which has swollen or is likely to become swollen.

## Equipment
*a)*  Soap and water.
*b)*  A length of ribbon, 1cm width.
*c)*  Ring-cutters.
*d)*  Feeler-gauges.
*e)*  Two pairs of Spencer-Wells forceps.

## Procedure
1  Explain the successive procedures to the patient.
2  Position the patient in comfort with the affected hand exposed.

### A  SOAP AND WATER METHOD
3  Apply cold soapy water to the finger and try to remove the ring by twisting. The patient may find it easier to do this himself.

### B  RIBBON METHOD
4  Slide about 5cm of ribbon underneath the ring, from the finger-tip side to the hand side, using a feeler-gauge if necessary.
5  Wind the long end of the ribbon (the finger-tip end) tightly around the finger, overlapping each turn, until the knuckle is completely covered. (Figure **245**)
6  Grip the short end of the ribbon (the hand end) and gently unwind the ribbon, applying traction to the ribbon in the direction of the finger-tip.
7  The ring should slide towards the finger-tip. (Figure **246**). Steps 4 to 7 can be repeated, if necessary.

### C  RING-CUTTERS METHOD
8  Obtain the patient's written permission to remove the ring by cutting it.
9  Position the hand, palm upwards, on a firm surface. Select the cutting site carefully in order to damage the ring as little as possible. (Figure **247**)
10  Slip the foot of the ring-cutters under the ring. Because heat is produced by the action of the blade, it is advisable to place a feeler-gauge underneath the ring-cutters to protect the finger. (Figure **248**)
11  Apply firm pressure to the handles and twist the blade. (Figure **249**)
12  When the ring has been cut through (Figure **250**), use Spencer-Wells forceps to separate and gently ease the ring off the finger. (Figure **251**)
13  It may be necessary to cut the ring in half.

**245**

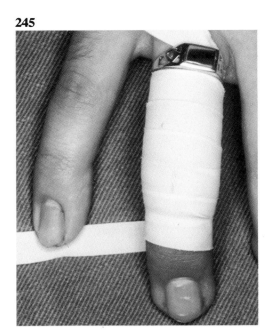

**246**

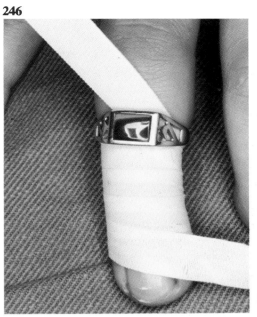

**247**

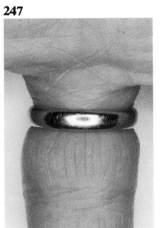

**248**

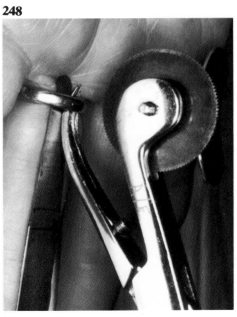

**249**

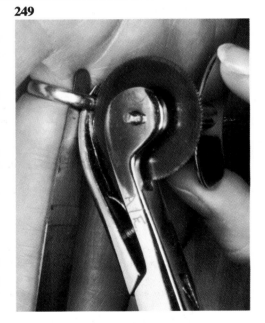

**250**

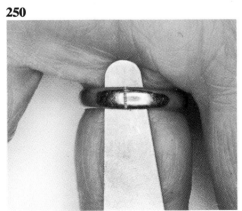

**251**

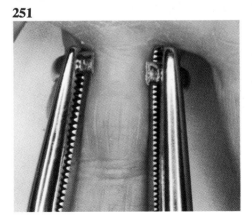

# 76 Nail trephining

## Use
To release blood from under the nail (subungual haematoma).

## Equipment
a) Sterile dressing pack, comprising:
   Four pairs of non-toothed forceps
   Gallipot
   Paper towels
   Gauze
   Cotton wool balls
   Tray
b) Spirit lamp.
c) Box of matches.
d) Paper clip.
e) Fire-proof safety mat.
f) Cleansing solution.

## Procedure
1 Explain the procedure to the patient.
2 Position the patient lying down in comfort, with his hand, palm downwards, on a firm surface. (Figure 252)
3 Clean the nail with cleansing solution.
4 Put the spirit lamp on the fire-proof mat and light the lamp.
5 Straighten out the paper clip, hold it in a piece of gauze and heat the tip in the flame until it becomes red hot.
6 Apply the red hot tip of the paper clip to the central point of the subungual haematoma (Figure 253). It will burn a hole in the nail through which blood will escape. (Figure 254)
7 Squeeze the area to express the blood.
8 Apply a finger dressing (see page 66).

## Advice to patients
Keep the dressing in place for about two days.

**252**

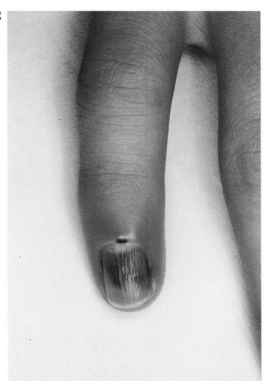

**253**

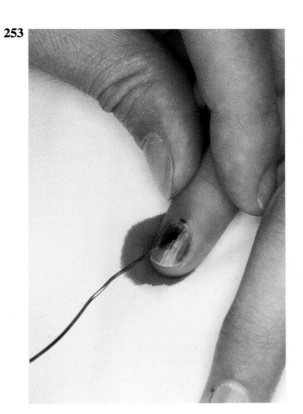

**254**

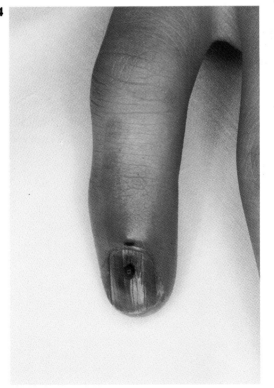

# 77 Intramuscular injection

## Use
To inject a drug into a muscle.

## Equipment
a) Syringe, large enough for the volume of drug to be given.
b) Two sterile needles, 21 gauge.
c) Alcohol-impregnated swabs.
d) The prescribed drug, together with the correct fluid in which to dissolve it if necessary, and the relevant prescription sheet. (Two nurses, one of whom is qualified, must check that the drug and the dose are correct according to the prescription sheet.)

## Procedure
1 Explain the procedure to the patient. Position him lying down in comfort on his side and expose his buttock or thigh.
2 Draw up the correct dose of the drug, dissolving it in fluid if necessary. Change the needle on the syringe and expel any air from the syringe.
3 Swab the area to be injected: this is usually either the upper outer quadrant of the buttock or the outer aspect of the upper third of the thigh.
4 Introduce the needle like a dart, at right angles to the skin, almost to the hilt of the needle in an average adult. (Figure 255)
5 Withdraw the plunger of the syringe slightly, to ensure the needle is not in a blood vessel. If no blood appears, inject the drug. (Figure 256)
6 Place a swab over the injection site and remove the needle quickly and in a straight line: Swab the site.
7 Sign the prescription sheet, to show that the drug has been given. Record the time.


*N.B.* Two drugs should not be injected at the same site, unless the doctor instructs otherwise.

## Advice to patients
If the area becomes red or swollen, return to hospital.

**255**

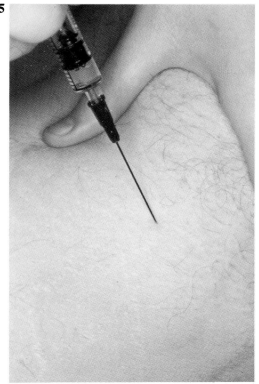

**256**

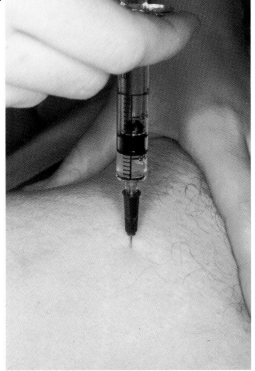

# 78 Subcutaneous injection

## Use
To inject a drug under the skin.

## Equipment
a) Syringe, large enough for the volume of drug to be given.
b) Sterile needle, 21 gauge.
c) Sterile needle, 25 gauge.
d) Alcohol-impregnated swabs.
e) The prescribed drug, together with the correct fluid in which to dissolve it if necessary, and the relevant prescription sheet. (Two nurses, one of whom is qualified, must check that the drug and the dose are correct according to the prescription sheet.)

## Procedure
1 Explain the procedure to the patient. Position him lying down or sitting in comfort. Expose the area selected for injection.
2 Use a 21 gauge needle to draw up the correct dose of the drug, dissolving it in fluid if necessary. Change to a 25 gauge needle and expel any air from the syringe.
3 Swab the area to be injected: common sites include the outer aspect of the upper arm, the outer aspect of the thigh or the abdominal wall below the umbilicus.
4 Pinch up the skin between your finger and thumb, swab the skin, and introduce the needle at an angle of about 20°, almost to the hilt of the needle. (Figure 257)
5 Withdraw the plunger of the syringe slightly, to ensure the needle is not in a blood vessel. If no blood appears, inject the drug. (Figure 258)
6 Place a swab over the injection site and remove the needle quickly and in a straight line. Swab the site.
7 Sign the prescription sheet, to show that the drug has been given. Record the time.

## Advice to patients
If the area becomes red or swollen, return to hospital.

**257**

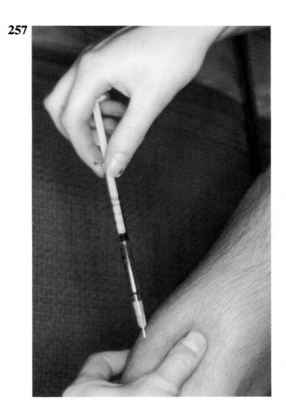

**258**

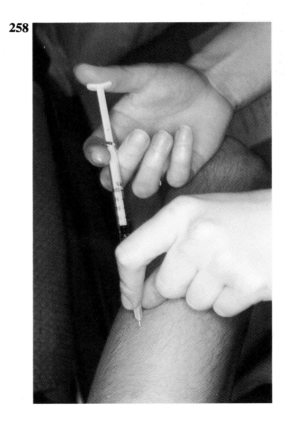

# 79 E.C.G. Recordings

## Use
To record the electrical activity of the heart.

## Equipment
a) Electrocardiograph (E.C.G.) machine, fitted with sufficient paper.
b) Electrode gel.
c) Four wrist/ankle bracelets.
d) Chest sucker.
e) Tissues.
f) Razor.

N.B. Various E.C.G. machines are available and each have instruction manuals, which provide details for recording the E.C.G.

A standard E.C.G. consists of twelve leads:
  three bipolar leads (I, II, III);
  three unipolar limb leads (aVr, aVl, aVf);
  six unipolar chest leads (V1, V2, V3, V4, V5, V6).

Normally, an E.C.G. is recorded at a rate of 25mm per second. The E.C.G. paper is printed with thin vertical lines 1mm apart (representing 0.04 seconds) and thick vertical lines 5mm apart (representing 0.2 seconds).

## Procedure
1 Explain the procedure to the patient and ask him to lie as still as possible during the recording.
2 Position the patient lying down in comfort. Remove all jewellery from wrists and ankles.
3 Undress the patient to the waist. Shave the chest if necessary, where the chest sucker is to be applied. Expose the ankles.
4 Smear some electrode gel on to each bracelet and attach a bracelet to each wrist and each ankle.
5 Connect each limb lead to the correct limb bracelet: each of the five leads (right arm, left arm, right leg, left leg, chest) is identified either by colour or markings.
6 Ensure a working power source, either mains or battery, is available.
7 Switch on the machine.
8 Set the sensitivity, centralise the stylus and calibrate the machine, according to the instruction manual.
9 Write the patient's name, the date and the time on the E.C.G. paper.
10 Record, one by one, leads I, II, III, aVr, aVl, aVf, according to the instruction manual. Record at least four full beats of the heart for each lead. Mark where each lead begins on the E.C.G. paper.
11 Attach the chest sucker to the correct lead (i.e. the only one of the five which is still unconnected).

12 Spread electrode gel at the following sites (Figure **259**):
  (a) 4th intercostal space just to the right of the sternum (V1);
  (b) 4th intercostal space just to the left of the sternum (V2);
  (c) midway between V2 and V4 (V3);
  (d) 5th intercostal space in the left midclavicular line (V4);
  (e) left anterior axillary line at the same horizontal level as V4 (V5);
  (f) left mid-axillary line at the same horizontal level as V4 (V6).
13 Attach the chest sucker to the V1 position and record lead V1, according to the instruction manual. Record at least four full beats of the heart. Mark where V1 begins on the E.C.G. paper.
14 Repeat step 13 for each of the other five chest leads (V2, V3, V4, V5, V6).
15 Switch off the machine.
16 Remove the chest sucker and the four bracelets from the patient and wipe off the electrode gel with tissues. Make the patient comfortable.
17 Clean any electrode gel off the bracelets and leave the equipment clean and tidy.

**259**

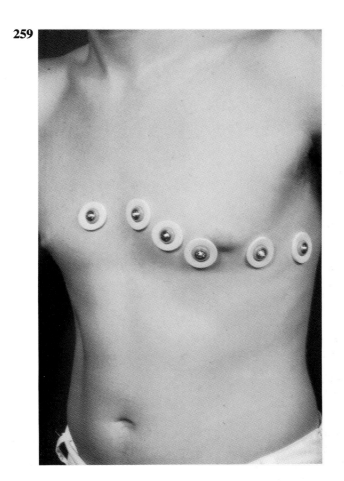

# 80 Gastric lavage

## Use
To empty the stomach.

## Equipment
a) Trolley, which can be tipped into a head-down position.
b) Large bowl, filled with luke-warm water.
c) Measuring jug.
d) Bucket.
e) Gastric tube.
f) Funnel, tubing and connections.
g) Litmus paper.
h) Incontinence sheets.
i) Denture pot.
j) Specimen jar and laboratory request forms.
k) Gown and paper cap for the patient.
l) Aprons and overshoes for the nurses.
m) Oxygen and suction must be readily available.

## Procedure
N.B. If the patient is unconscious, an anaesthetist is required to pass the gastric tube, as the gag reflex may be absent and the patient may need an endotracheal tube prior to gastric lavage. Two nurses are needed.

1  Explain the procedure to the patient.
2  Record the patient's temperature, pulse rate, respiratory rate, blood pressure, colour and conscious level.
3  Undress the patient and put into a gown and paper cap. Place any dentures in a labelled denture pot. Remove jewellery and store with the patient's property.
4  Position the patient on a trolley lying on his right side.
5  Remove any pillows and place an incontinence sheet under the patient's head.
6  Put the bucket on the floor at the head of the trolley.
7  Tip the trolley head down.
8  Pass the gastric tube through the patient's mouth smoothly and firmly, asking the patient to swallow as you do so. (Figure **260**)
9  When the gastric tube reaches the stomach, aspirate should come through the tube and into the bucket, indicating that the tube is correctly situated.
10  Test the aspirate with blue litmus paper: the acid from the stomach turns it red.
11  If the tube remains empty, check that the patient's colour remains satisfactory: if cyanosis develops, the tube may be in the lungs and must be repositioned.

12  When you are satisfied that the gastric tube is correctly positioned in the stomach, connect the funnel and tubing to the gastric tube.
13  Ask the patient to breathe slowly through his mouth.
14  Fill the funnel with 200ml of luke-warm water, using a measuring jug. Raise the funnel high into the air until all the water passes down the tube into the stomach. (Figure **261**)
15  Lower the funnel to the ground to allow the water and stomach contents to flow back into the funnel. Empty the contents into the bucket, ensuring that at least 200ml is returned. (Figure **262**)
16  Continue until the water coming back is clear, using 500ml of water each time. Ensure that the volume being returned is equal to or greater than the volume being introduced.
17  It may be necessary to apply suction to the patient's mouth to clear secretions as the procedure continues.
18  Disconnect the funnel and tubing from the gastric tube.
19  Gently but firmly remove the gastric tube.
20  Position the patient in comfort and again record his temperature, pulse rate, respiratory rate, blood pressure, colour and conscious level.
21  Record the contents of the gastric aspirate and send a sample in a specimen jar for laboratory analysis, if required.

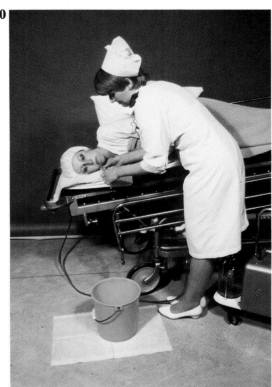

260

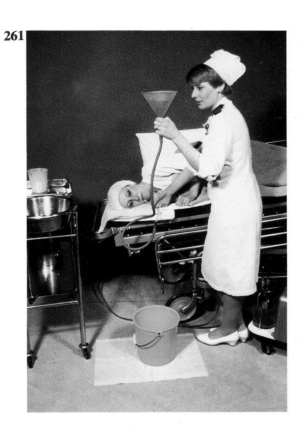

261

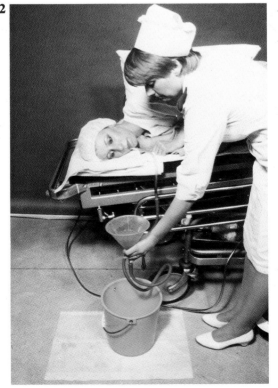

262

# Index

Figures in light type refer to pages; those in **bold** type refer to illustrations.

Povidone-iodi
Proflavine *c*
Pus, *see l*